YORKSHIRE AND
OF MEDI(

Front cover: *Sir Arthur Mayo-Robson, surgeon to The General Infirmary at Leeds 1884-1902. (By kind permission of the Special Trustees of the Infirmary).*

Back cover: *Sir James Crichton-Browne, Director of the West Riding Lunatic Asylum where Ferrier did his work on cerebral localisation. (By kind permission of the Royal College of Physicians).*

For
W.K.M.
in recognition of his many services to
The Medical School at Leeds
and
The Yorkshire Medical and Dental History Society.

YORKSHIRE
AND THE
HISTORY OF MEDICINE

Malcolm Parsons
Formerly Consultant Neurologist at
The General Infirmary at Leeds and
Pinderfields Hospital Wakefield

William Sessions Limited
York, England

© Dr Malcolm Parsons 2002

ISBN 1 85072 273 0

Printed in 11 on 12 point Plantin Typeface
from Author's Disk
by Sessions of York
The Ebor Press
York, England

Contents

Chapter		Page
	Preface	viii
I	Rome and the Monastic Foundations	1
II	Religio Medici – the Halifax Connection	9
III	Quakers	14
IV	Facts and Fevers	25
V	Medical Artists	31
VI	Psychiatry	39
VII	'A Scientific Phrenology'	47
VIII	Industrial Medicine	56
IX	The Leeds Anatomy Riots – 1832	63
X	The Development of Anaesthesia	72
XI	The General Infirmary at Leeds	78
XII	The Development of Surgery at Leeds	85
XIII	Clifford Allbutt and the Development of Modern Medicine	97
XIV	The Lessons of History	106
	Glossary	109

Illustrations

		Page
Fig. 1a,b	Panels from the St. William's Window in York Minster	5
Fig. 2.	The invasion of the College of Physicians in Warwick Lane	18
Fig. 3.	Fleet Street looking west	19
Fig. 4.	Engravings prepared by George Stubbs for John Burton's treatise on obstetrics	35
Fig. 5.	John Burton's memorial in Holy Trinity, Micklegate, York	37
Fig. 6.	The laboratory at Stanley Royd Hospital, Wakefield	52
Fig. 7.	The grave of Charles Turner Thackrah	62
Fig. 8.	Cartoon of the banner carried at the election in Leeds 1832	71
Fig. 9.	A bird's-eye view of the General Infirmary at Leeds, 1869	81
Fig. 10.	Stonework on the General Infirmary at Leeds	81
Fig. 11.	A design, drawn up in 1910, which would have provided the General Infirmary at Leeds with six identical ward blocks along the south front	83

Fig. 12.	One of the twin theatres in the General Infirmary at Leeds, built in 1897	92
Fig. 13.	A view of the old theatre block at the General Infirmary at Leeds	94
Fig. 14.	Allbutt's thermometer	99
Fig. 15.	'Moynihan's pond'	105

Preface

ACCOUNTS OF THE history of medicine, of which there are many, tend to concentrate on events in major centres such as London and Edinburgh and to forget the birthplaces of leading figures and the efforts of those who worked in the provinces. This book is an attempt, where Yorkshire is concerned, to redress the balance. Taking a series of topics of local interest from the last 2,000 years I have tried, in simple language, to set them in the context of the times. In this way I hope, without attempting to give a heavy, comprehensive survey, to convey a feeling of the various periods and to draw attention to some of their main characters and events. The book makes no claim to originality or scholarship, as for the most part I am simply repeating stories that have already been told elsewhere. These articles, however, are often in relatively obscure journals, and for this reason in addition to giving the main references I have quoted extensively from them. In this way I hope to arouse interest in a somewhat neglected topic and to encourage those who are better informed to correct errors or omissions, so that the medical history of this great county can be properly recorded.

I would like to express my thanks to Professor Sir Christopher Booth of the Wellcome Trust Centre for the History of Medicine for the interest he has taken in this project, for his detailed comments on the manuscript and for his encouragement and advice. In attempting to survey this vast subject it has been most reassuring to have the support of the leading authority on the history of medicine in Yorkshire.

M.P. January 2002.

CHAPTER I

Rome and the Monastic Foundations

The Christian church, which played so great a part in the development of English medicine, is perhaps the most neglected relic of the Roman occupation.

THOSE PERPLEXED by the origins of English medicine will find in the vicinity of York Minster four objects to guide their thoughts. The first is the Saint William's window in the Minster, which speaks of the spiritual healing so important to the medieval church. The second is St. Peter's School near Bootham Bar, a reminder of the Northumbrian ecclesiastical scholarship which anticipated early western universities like Salerno by two centuries. The third is the ruins of St. Leonard's Hospital in the museum gardens - a relic of the care which the church provided for the sick and needy throughout the darkest days of English history. And the fourth, outside the south door of the Minster, is a Roman emperor.

The statue of **Constantine the Great** (c274-337) commemorates his proclamation as Emperor by his troops in York in AD 306, and it is not immediately apparent what bearing it has on the history of medicine. He was, of course, a representative of the power that brought civilisation (and organised medicine) to these hitherto barbaric islands. But medicine was not one of Rome's great strengths and Romans, who retained an enduring respect for traditional, supernatural methods, did not regard the discipline as a suitable occupation for a Roman citizen. They were however prepared to accept the services of Greek physicians who prospered and, with the expansion of the Empire, spread their ideas throughout the then-known world. From a practical point of view this was of little value, for their knowledge of the subject was limited. It did however result in a lucrative (and corrupt) trade in pharmaceuticals, of which a pot marked 'Ex radice Britanica' (sic) - thought to have contained dock for the treatment of scurvy - is an interesting relic. It also led to developments in the one area in which the Romans excelled - the provision of military hospitals.

For an army of occupation sick and injured soldiers posed a difficult problem, as it was clearly impossible to adopt the usual policy of billeting them on the civilian population. But keeping casualties in the same quarters as their colleagues had a demoralising effect on those who were fit, and for this reason it was customary to provide military bases with hospitals like the one at Housesteads in Northumberland - perhaps the earliest example of organised medicine in the country. These well-planned hospitals were staffed by army surgeons or *medici* whose instruments (examples of which have been found) were sometimes depicted on their gravestones. It was presumably one such who operated on the skull exhumed from the Roman cemetery in York which shows clear evidence of having been opened with a trephine. It is moreover probable that Roman surgeons who left the army but continued to live in Britain were the prototype of the first English physician, the Anglo-Saxon *leche* (the word from which the surname Leach is derived). Certainly **Wycliffe** (a Yorkshireman) used the word *leche* for *medicus* when translating the Vulgate into the vernacular at the end of the 14th century.

Indirectly, however, Constantine made a second and even greater contribution to English medicine, for he was the Emperor who adopted Christianity as the official religion of the Empire. The benefits of this policy, however, were not immediately apparent. Indeed, despite Augustine's assertion in his book *De civitate Dei* (The City of God) that the disasters about to occur were a penalty for past sins, it seemed to many that they were a consequence of deserting the traditional gods. Be that as it may, shortly afterwards the Western half of the now divided Empire collapsed, its provinces were abandoned and in 476 Rome itself fell to the barbarians. For Europe, which lapsed into a chaos of warring states, it was an unmitigated disaster that destroyed all semblance of civilisation and reduced once-great cities like London to ghost towns.

The 'Christian Empire'

It was in 596, amidst these unpromising circumstances, that pope Gregory the Great conceived the idea of a new, spiritual empire of which he, *servus servorum dei*, was to be the head. So, in the words of Bryant, 'as panic-stricken bureaucrats abandoned the frontiers province after province, Christian missionaries, resuming the mission the Caesars had abandoned, carried the faith into the forest stockades and nomad camps of the barbarians.' It was, in truth, a primitive form of Christianity which they implanted. But pagan rulers were impressed by the gallantry of these ambassadors from a once-great Empire and attracted by a faith that held an answer to the horrors of the after-life. The mission, moreover, was not without local support for the remnants of the Christian communities deserted by the legions, which had taken refuge in Ireland and on the western fringes of the country, had started to return to Scotland and to Northumbria (England north of the Humber). Overcoming their initial suspicions these groups now re-united with Gregory's missionaries at the Synod of Whitby (664), forming a church whose activities in Europe were eventually to produce a 'Christian' empire even larger than its 'military' predecessor.

Barbarian rulers were quick to realise that these missionaries had more to offer than spiritual gifts. Unlike their hosts they could read and write and they were imbued with a passion for order and discipline. They had in Latin a common language and they were part of an international network that stretched across Europe. They were therefore ideally qualified to undertake the tasks of keeping records, administering the state and communicating with neighbouring countries. Indeed during the 7th century, as Europe descended into chaos, Northumbria (of which York was the chief city) became a political and academic centre of some significance. Its kings exercised suzerainty over the other kingdoms of England and the library at Jarrow, to which cartloads of books had been brought from Rome and Gaul, was reputed to be the largest in Europe. Clergy from the region travelled widely, exchanging ideas, and Bede (673-735) in particular was held to be the foremost scholar of his time. Far from being a backwater on the fringes of the Empire, it is known that in the 9th. century scholars in Northumbria were studying books which did not appear in Salerno (one of the first universities in Europe) for another two centuries. England was indeed the only country in Europe to have a medical literature in its native language, exemplified by the famous Leechbook of Bald. It was not therefore surprising that in the 8th century, when Charlemagne (who could not himself read or write) decided to promote a revival of learning in Europe, he chose **Alcuin** (732-804), a priest from York, as his adviser.

Being at once the spiritual and the academic centre of the state it was inevitable that people should turn to the Church in times of sickness. There were three reasons for this. First and foremost it was an <u>age of faith</u>, an age in which the main consideration - for both priest and people - was that a patient should die in a state of grace. But it was a faith which owed more than a little to its pagan ancestors, for the charms and rituals associated with the collection of herbs and prayers of healing had been retained as a direct result of Gregory's advice that pagan sites and practices should be assimilated into Christian worship. This policy was most evident in the vast array of relics (bits of saints, their clothing or possessions) kept, to their great financial advantage, in the churches, for close contact with such objects was supposed to expose the suppliant to a powerful healing force.

Most important of these relics were the shrines, usually found in cathedrals, which contained the entire body of a saint. Set on pillars behind the high altar, these richly decorated caskets (of which the Confessor's shrine in Westminster Abbey is the only one to survive) were widely venerated. As in the Greek Aesculapia, it was customary for suppliants to leave before them wax models of defective limbs or organs and to burn candles made of waxed bandages which had been bound round the affected part.[1] York, not to be out-done by Becket's tomb at Canterbury, had its own shrine of this sort, dedicated to **St. William**. William Fitzherbert, the great grandson of William the Conqueror, had been created Archbishop of York in 1141 but was immediately expelled by the pope on the grounds that the king had influenced his appointment. Although subsequently restored to office he died three weeks later, having being taken ill suddenly (and possibly poisoned) while celebrating mass. In that short time, however, he was credited with a number of miracles and his shrine (which was demolished in the Reformation) soon became a place of pilgrimage. Although only fragments of the shrine have survived illustrations of it can be seen, along with scenes from William's life, of the miracles he performed and of the models and candles brought by suppliants, in the 15th century St. William's window on the north side of the Minster choir (Figs. 1a & 1b).

In addition to being men of faith, however, the clergy were also <u>men of learning</u> - such men as might be expected to know how to

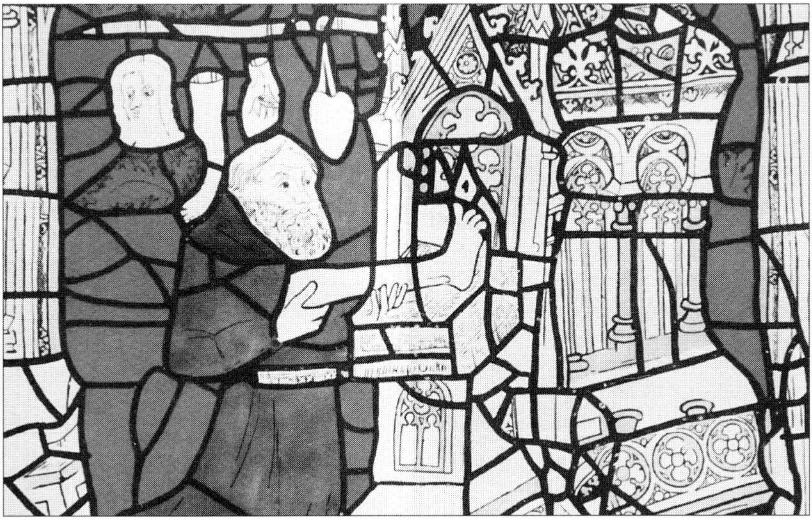

Fig. 1a. Panel from the St. William's Window in York Minster, showing wax models of limbs, hearts etc being offered before St. William's shrine.
(By kind permission of the Dean and Chapter)

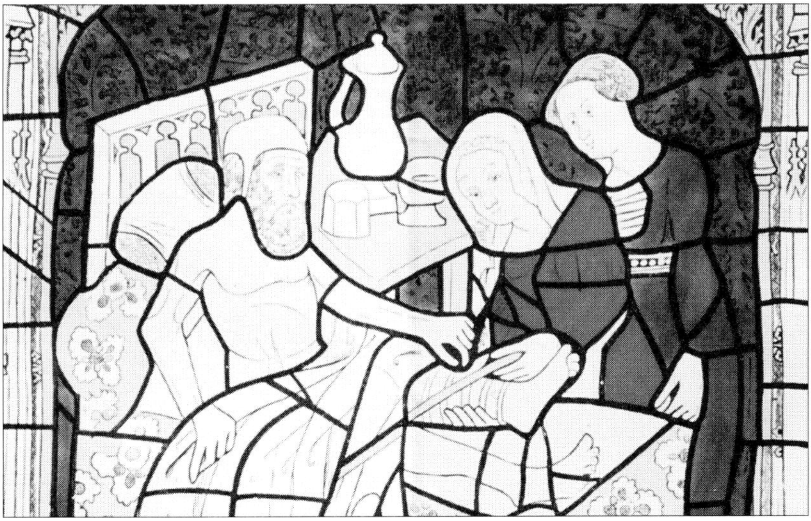

Fig. 1b. Panel from the St. William's window in York Minster showing an injured limb being bound in waxed tape that would later be formed into a votive candle.
(By kind permission of the Dean and Chapter)

deal with illness or injury. Most religious houses had an *infirmarius* and if that did not suffice they were happy - once the safety of the patient's soul had been ensured - to enlist the aid of a leech. Some monasteries even had physicians on the staff and occasionally, as in the case of **Paulinus**,[2] master of St. Leonard's Hospital York in 1155, the physician was himself a priest. It is by no means clear what training and qualifications these early physicians had, for it was not until the 14th century that the Universities and the Company of Barber Surgeons appeared with their different but clearly defined methods of instruction and assessment. Nevertheless scholars such as Columba and Bede acquired a profound knowledge of medicine, for their writings contain accounts of the four humours, detailed descriptions of patients, instructions on the letting of blood and notes on the healing properties of herbs. This interest was evidently shared by many others, for in 1130 the Council of Clermont had to impose a ban on regular clergy leaving their monasteries to obtain training in medicine - a measure which was clearly ineffective, for in 1478 a later pope had to issue another edict absolving those who did. There was however no objection to them leaving their monasteries to *practice* medicine - a fact which the monk Simon of Ryedale turned to good advantage when, having cured the wife of William de Tanton, he went on to have an affair with her.

The Church's third contribution, which to many was more important than its spiritual and medical care, was the provision of hospitals. For the most part these were not hospitals in the modern sense for, like the great hospitals of Revolutionary Paris, they were mainly designed for the outcasts in society - to sustain, as one statute put it, 'impotent Men and Women, Lazars, Men out of their Wits and poor Women with child'. English hospitals were smaller than their Continental counterparts and many concentrated on one particular group - lepers, the insane or (as in the case of the Rerecross on the remote Richmond-Carlisle road) travellers. In most, the care of the sick and injured seems to have been of secondary importance. In this respect St. Leonard's Hospital at York was an exception. Originally called St. Peter's after the Minster to which it was attached, it was probably founded in the 10th century. One of the largest (and oldest) hospitals in the country, some of its 200 beds were occupied by people who had bought *corrodies* or *liveries* - a sort of medieval longterm care plan. Others were supported, at the expense of the hospital, in *cremettal* beds and in addition food was distributed to regular and casual 'outpatients', to four leper hospitals and to the prisoners in York Castle. St. Leonard's, like St. Bartholomew's (a very similar Augustinian foundation) was however unusual in that it also catered for those with acute illnesses who, according to the statutes, were not to be discharged until they were fit to work.

These hospitals, which provided a vital medical and social service to the community, were soon to encounter two disasters. The first, in the 14th century, was the Black Death which decimated the population and greatly reduced the income of the religious foundations. Many failed to survive and such as did had to curtail their activities. To some extent this deficit was made good by wealthy merchants and guilds who founded numerous establishments which were in effect alms houses. Most, like William Browne's Hospital at Stamford, were small, had no medical facilities and offered no 'outpatient' services. Browne's hospital simply provided housing for twelve poor, ten men and two women, the latter - as the charter craftily specifies - ' to have special care of the men when they become sick, weak or helpless'. Being poorly endowed, many such hospitals failed to survive.

The second disaster, which occurred a century later, was the dissolution of the monasteries by Henry VIII - a measure which instantly deprived the country of most of its hospital and social services. London, once 'a city of palaces', became 'a city of ruins' and even the king was alarmed to find how the streets filled with 'lazars and the lame'. Ordered to resolve the matter the Lord Mayor, Sir Richard Gresham, contrived to obtain five Royal Hospitals. This was no great act of charity on the part of the monarch, for four of them had just been stolen and the fifth - the old Bridewell Palace - was 'no longer liked on account of the fylthy stynkyng dytch (the Fleet River, which contained all the rubbish from Smithfield) which runneth along the side of it'. But the damage was not confined to London. York, with its assembly of Augustinian, Benedictine, Dominican, Carmelite and Franciscan houses was devastated, as was the surrounding countryside where abbeys like Bolton, Byland, Fountains, Jervaulx, Kirkstall, Rievaulx and Selby were an essential part, not only of the religious and social life of the community but also of the economy. It was the destruction of these religious foundations that was largely responsible for the Pilgrimage of Grace. But despite this protest the majority of England was less fortunate than London, and apart from the parish workhouse it was to be left without a 'hospital' service for two centuries, when once more a (largely nonconformist) religious movement was heavily involved in the foundation of civic dispensaries and hospitals.

REFERENCES

Cullum, P.H. Cremetts and Corrodies: Care of the Poor and Sick at St. Leonard's Hospital York in the Middle Ages. University of York Borthwick Papers No. 79.

Fowler, J. St. William's Window. Yorkshire Archaeological and Topographical Journal 1874.3.198.

Gardner, R. Medicine in Anglo-Saxon Northumbria in Medicine in Northumbria. Pybus Society 1993.

Griffin, J.P. London's Medieval Hospitals and the Reformation. Journal of the Royal College of Physicians 1998.32.72.

Stell, P. Medical Practice in Medieval York. University of York Borthwick Papers No. 90.

NOTES

1. These traditions account for the close relationship between the Guild of Chandlers and the Guild of Barber Surgeons, both of whom used wax - to prepare ointments and to manufacture votive models and candles.
2. Paulinus, the first *medicus* in York who is known by name, went on to become Vicar of Leeds.

CHAPTER II

Religio Medici – the Halifax Connection

The training of a 17th century physician was not designed to impart a knowledge of medicine (of which there was little) but to produce a man of culture. It is for this attribute that they are often remembered.

TO WILLIAM OSLER, **Thomas Browne** (1605-1682) was an icon. His admiration was not, however, based on Browne's clinical abilities, for a physician who appeared for the prosecution in the trial of two witches is unlikely to appeal to the Regius Professor of Medicine at Oxford. Rather it depended on his authorship 'for my private exercise and satisfaction' of a little book called *Religio Medici*. First appearing in an unauthorised form in 1642, this physician's *credo* which, as Osler put it, 'mingles the waters of science with the oil of faith', was to become a devotional classic.

Osler was introduced to *Religio Medici* at the age of 16. He bought the 1862 edition - the second book in his vast library - when he was 18 and referred to and recommended it throughout his long life. He collected all but one of the 55 editions and translations (a 1688 Dutch version) and in due course brought out his own edition, set in the beautiful type designed by Bishop Fell (Willis' father-in-law) in 1660 -'perhaps the oldest font in use in England'. Of all his books it was clearly the one most dear to him and it was in recognition of this fact that, at his funeral in Christ Church Cathedral, Oxford on January 1st. 1920, the 1862 edition he had bought 52 years earlier was placed on his coffin.

It was of course inevitable that Osler's interest should extend from the book to its author and when he was 23 he visited Norwich, where Browne spent most of his life. He went to see his resting places - two of them, for during repairs to St. Peter Mancroft in 1840 Browne's grave had been opened and the skull had been removed. This was ironical, for in another of his books, *Urn Burial*, Browne himself spoke of the 'tragic abomination of being knaved out of our graves' and asked 'who knows the fate of his bones or how often he is to be buried?'. Osler was distressed to find the skull on display in the museum of the Norfolk and Norwich Hospital and twenty-eight years later he provided a suitable container in the form of an engraved casket made by the Goldsmiths' and Silversmiths' Company. He was also instrumental in the erection of a statue, unveiled in 1905, but he did not live to see the skull restored to the grave in 1922.

Despite his almost obsessional interest in Browne and his works, Osler appears to have taken little interest in his early life. This is strange, for one of the two things we know with certainty about the writing of *Religio Medici* is that it was done 'before my pulse hath beat 30 years'. Browne was born in London in 1605 and was educated at Winchester and Pembroke College Oxford. It is generally agreed that he then spent several years on the Continent, obtaining an M.D. at Leiden in 1633 (although, as Osler discovered, there is no record of this in the University archives). This, however, did not entitle him to practise without supervision in England until his degree had been 'incorporated' by his own University. There was therefore a gap of four years between his return from Leiden and his appearance in Norwich in 1637, and passages in the book show that it was during this time that *Religio Medici* was written. But where was this done?

There appear to be two answers to this question. The first, attributed to the Oxford antiquarian Anthony Wood, suggests that Browne 'Practiced for some time in Oxfordshire'. This would make sense, for he had friends at Oxford and might well have worked under the supervision of an older physician while he waited for his degree to be incorporated. But although Wood had a considerable knowledge of Oxford society neither he nor Aubrey (from whom he obtained much of his information) knew Browne personally, for they were only five and eleven years old when he moved to Norwich. Moreover, if one looks carefully at Wood's original statement[1] it actually says that Browne practised in Oxford *before* going to Leiden. He says nothing of what happened between 1633 and 1637 when he 'retired to Norwich.' But an even more telling argument against the 'Oxford solution' is the second undisputed fact about the production of the book. This, again, is Browne's own statement that 'It was penned in such a place and with such disadvantage that (I protest) from the first setting of pen unto paper I had not the assistance of any good book whereby to promote my invention or relieve my memory'. Such a remark is surely incompatible with a University city or its environs.

The alternative suggestion is that the book was written in Shibden Dale, which lies between Halifax and Bradford. This idea was first put forward in a book entitled *Halifax and its Gibbet Law*, published in 1708 by William Bentley, clerk to Halifax Parish Church. The author, however, was a local medical practitioner called Samuel Midgley who was incarcerated in Halifax jail for debt. Like Wood and Aubrey, Midgley was only seven when Browne moved to Norwich, but he is unequivocal in listing among 'the physicians and professors in that science' who had worked in the locality 'the learned Dr. Browne, because in his juvenal years he fixed himself in this populous and rich trading place, wherein to show his skill and to gain respect in the world, and that during his residence among us in his vacant hours he writ his admired piece called by him *Religio Medici*'. This suggests that, while he was waiting for his degree to be incorporated, Browne continued to practise as a physician out of sight of the none-too-vigilant authorities. When, subsequently, he became famous, his name would no doubt have been mentioned in Midgley's hearing by his fellow practitioners.

Thirty years later, in a book entitled *Antiquities of the Parish of Halifax* (1738) Thomas Wright, a curate at the Parish Church, confirmed that Browne 'practised here as a physician in his younger days' (although he gives an incorrect date - 1630) and goes on to specify that he lived at Shipden Hall. Unfortunately this information, while strengthening the overall case for Halifax, raises another problem, for over the years Halifax has had several buildings of that name. We can clearly exclude the well-known (Lower) Shibden Hall, now a museum, for at the material time that was in the hands of a family called Lister. We can also exclude the present Upper Shibden Hall, a burnt-out ruin near Catherine Slack, for this was only built in about 1820 by Michael Stocks, a brewer and colliery owner who owned the Upper Shibden estate. Moreover, until about 1900 this building was known as Catherine Hall, for there was on the estate the remains of another, much older, Upper Shibden Hall - the one in which Browne lived.

This building was one of a number of old timber-framed houses in the vicinity that were renovated in the 17th century. There do not appear to be any pictures of it and the only description of it comes from the Rev. Bryan Dale - a student of Thomas Browne - who visited it towards the end of the 19th century. He tells us that the Hall - by then converted into a farmhouse - stood 'high on a hill overlooking the valley'. It had 'a double porch of hewn stone and a carved oak ceiling'. But the occupant, a tenant of Michael Stocks, was under notice to quit and when Dale published his account in 1896 the Hall had been 'taken down and replaced by two cottages'.[2] It was presumably at this stage that Catherine Hall assumed the name of Upper Shibden Hall.

Even today, the site of Browne's Upper Shibden Hall is well outside Halifax and, unlike Oxford, is in keeping with his claim that he 'had not the assistance of any good book'. But Dale made one further observation that lends support to the story that this was once Browne's home. Over the fireplace were carved the initials 'JSF' and the date 1626. These were the initials of James Foxcroft and of his wife Sarah who effected the renovation. Foxcroft did not live in his house for long, however, for by 1638 he was sufficiently well established in Halifax to appear on the list of City Constables as 'James Foxcroft of The Cross, formerly of Upper Shipden Hall'. The Hall may therefore have been vacant when Browne returned from the Continent. Indeed it is possible to work out how he might have discovered this, for James Foxcroft's brother Anthony was to marry the widow of one of Browne's friends, John Power. Moreover, after his move to Nottingham, Power's son Dr Henry Power (who has the distinction of being one of the first two people elected to the Royal Society) sent Browne 'three old Spanish books which once belonged to my father, who did much honour you' and passed on items of news which could only have been of interest to someone who knew the locality well.

While it is strange that we should have no concrete evidence of Browne's whereabouts at this crucial stage of his life there are, therefore, good reasons to believe the story that he was in Halifax. It was started by a member of the local medical community who was alive at the time. The house named was suitably remote and was probably vacant. The owner was distantly related to one of Browne's close friends. And the son of that friend continued to regale him with news of the locality after he moved to Norwich. It therefore seems that this little book which was written for friends, which became a classic, which inspired Osler throughout his life and which, two hundred years later, was to accompany him to his grave, was probably written in this remote Yorkshire valley. Osler, however, was by no means the first person to be inspired by it. To modern eyes the text is obscure, yet there is something familiar about the words and the cadence of the famous dormitive. Take the lines:

> Sleep is a death, O make me try
> By sleeping what it is to die
> And as gently lay my head
> On my grave, as on my bed.

Was it, as Osler himself asked, simply a coincidence that in his famous evening hymn Bishop Thomas Ken (1637-1711) wrote:

> Teach me to live that I may dread
> The grave as little as my bed.
> Teach me to die, that so I may
> Rise glorious at the awful day.

REFERENCES

Cushing, H. Life of Sir William Osler. Oxford 1925.
Dale, B. Shibden Dale and Sir Thomas Browne's 'Religio Medici'. Bradford Antiquary NS 1. 1896. 45.
Huntley, F.L. Sir Thomas Browne. Ann Arbor Press University of Michigan 1962.

NOTES

1. '... he took his degree in Arts as a Member of the said College, entered on the Physic line and practiced that Faculty for some time in these parts. Afterwards he travelled beyond the Seas, was made a Doctor of Physic at Leiden and after his return he was incorporated in the University in 1637. About that time he retired to Norwich'.
2. The grid reference on map 26 of the West Yorkshire Archaeological Survey to 1500 suggests that the Hall was a few yards south of a house called The Old Stables, which is near the present (ruined) Upper Shibden Hall.

CHAPTER III

Quakers

The practice as opposed to the science of medicine began to develop in the 18th century. This was in large measure due to activities of Quakers who, forced to train in the more modern schools at Leiden and Edinburgh, developed clinical methods and the dispensaries. Their contribution was not recognised by the College with whom they were in constant (and sometimes comical) conflict.

BY THE BEGINNING of the 18th century the control of medicine in England was firmly in the hands of the Royal College of Physicians. For all practical purposes this was a group of some 40 Fellows, society physicians who had trained at Oxford or Cambridge and were therefore, by definition, Anglicans. Although firmly convinced of their social and intellectual superiority their contributions to clinical medicine, to research and to teaching were in fact meagre.

Barely recognised by these luminaries was a second, much larger group of physicians who were, in many instances, better trained and more active than their colleagues in the College. Many were Scots from Edinburgh whose medical school, modelled on the great school at Leiden, was more clinically orientated than the two English universities. Others were Quakers, members of a vast and closely knit sect which, because of its reputation for industry and integrity, had become very influential. Unlike the academics in the English universities, from which they were excluded because of their faith, Quakers regarded abstract speculation as tantamount to idleness and concentrated on the practicalities of life. They were also unusual in that they had no sense of class and were eager to share their knowledge and to assist each other in every possible way. Above all, they were anxious to use their assets to improve society.[1]

Such men, for whom medicine was an ideal occupation, were well attuned to the practical training provided at Edinburgh and Leiden, and were destined to play a key role in the profession and in society.

Although Yorkshire was the home of many Quakers, the number of eminent physicians it produced is remarkable. Even more remarkable is the fact that many of them came from Wensleydale and the region round Sedbergh on the Yorkshire Westmorland border, an area which, even today, is one of the most remote and inaccessible parts of the English countryside. Hillary Hall at Burtersett, for example, was the home of **William Hillary** (1697-1763) whose book *Observations on the Changes of the Air and the Concomitant Epidemical Diseases in the Island of Barbados* is one of the first English textbooks on tropical diseases. It also contains the first account of tropical sprue. **Robert Willan** of Sedbergh (1757-1812), after whom the Willan Room in the College of Physicians is named, published the first great classification of diseases of the skin - work which was completed by his disciple and successor **Thomas Bateman** (1778-1821) of Whitby. The physician/savant John Dawson and his pupil John Haygarth, both from Wensleydale, and the Tukes of York will be mentioned in later chapters. But the two most illustrious Yorkshire Quakers, who founded important medical societies and, through the dispensary movement, brought medical care to the masses, were John Fothergill and John Coakley Lettsom.

John Fothergill (1712-1780)

John Fothergill was born at Carr End near Bainbridge in Wensleydale. Like several of his fellow Quakers he attended the famous local school at Sedbergh and was apprenticed to **Benjamin Bartlett**, a Quaker apothecary in Bradford. He then went to Edinburgh and to St. Thomas's in London, an excellent teaching hospital which had many Dissenters on its staff. He was the first Edinburgh graduate to become a Licentiate of the London College of Physicians, and although 'the pecuniary object of his calling was the last of his considerations', he developed a large and distinguished London practice whose patients included John Wesley, Clive of India and many leading politicians.

Medically Fothergill is remembered mainly for three things - his *Account of the Sore Throat Alternated with Ulcers* (based on an epidemic of diphtheria in 1747), his discovery of the cause of angina of effort and his description of trigeminal neuralgia. He also wrote on 'sick headache' (migraine) and on the problem of resuscitation, and it was on his orders that the Yorkshire physician **Nathaniel Hulme** (1732-1807) - who had himself been a mariner - provided Cook's ship the Endeavour with three 'mixes' of orange and lemon juice - part of a trial which established the value of fruit juice in the prevention of scurvy and was to earn Cook the Copley medal of the Royal Society. But Fothergill's interests extended far beyond medicine. He was an active member of the Society of Friends and was greatly concerned with social problems such as the condition of prisons, the widening of roads and the provision of burial grounds. He was an avid collector of shells, insects, minerals and documents - many of which passed after his death to William Hunter and thence to the museum in Glasgow. And he was an ardent botanist who corresponded with Linnaeus, had had a plant named after him and established a large botanical garden from which many rare specimens were sold to Catherine II of Russia after his death.

Fothergill also had an interest in politics, becoming involved in the contemporary dispute over the American colonies. This was a matter about which he was well informed, for he had relatives in America and was the London correspondent of the Society of Friends in Pennsylvania. Being convinced that the behaviour of the British government was both unreasonable and dangerous he did his utmost to bring about a reconciliation, a task which he was well qualified to undertake as he knew leading Americans such as Rush and Franklin and had among his English patients the Prime Minister, the Secretary of State for the American Colonies, the Speaker and the Lord Chancellor. Sadly his efforts were in vain and in due course his forebodings about the outcome proved to be correct.

The Society of Physicians

Fothergill's diplomacy was also needed in dealing with the affairs of his own profession which, at the time, was divided by several conflicts. Among other things, it was the duty of the College of Physicians to licence all those who practised medicine within seven miles of London - a regulation which was not very diligently enforced. It was however made abundantly clear to the Licentiates that they were only 'physicians to the lower orders'. As one dignitary succinctly explained, 'they (the Licentiates) stand in no other relationship to us (the Fellows) than the publican does to the bench of Justices from whom he receives a licence to sell beer.' The situation was in fact rather complicated. There was no denying that medical degrees from Aberdeen and Saint Andrew's, which could in effect be bought, were often worthless. On the other hand the highly esteemed qualifications from Oxford and Cambridge, although difficult to obtain, were also of little practical value. Graduates from Edinburgh, by contrast, had received as thorough a training in clinical medicine as was then available. Yet although these men, who included many of the most distinguished physicians in London, could obtain a Licence from the London College they were not allowed to participate in its activities. There was therefore more than a little truth in Fothergill's complaint that an organisation designed to support regular physicians and to suppress quackery had become 'a monopoly whose management had fallen into the hands of a few who raised themselves and laid others, no less knowing, able or honest, under great difficulties.'

This situation was deeply resented by the Licentiates who complained that the College, with its 'mouldering library and empty halls' had no interest in medicine. Attempts to participate in its management were, however, steadfastly resisted and eventually, to the delight of the general public, some of the bolder spirits smashed their way into the building in Warwick Lane and invaded its council chamber (Fig. 2). Fothergill's approach was less violent but more devastating. Realising that among the 'needy and half-educated adventurers' (ie Edinburgh graduates) the College was so anxious to exclude there were many of the most distinguished physicians in London he simply established a rival organisation 'for such as have the care of hospitals or are otherwise in some degree of repute in their profession.' Founded in 1752 the Medical Society, later known as the Society of Physicians, met in the Mitre Tavern[2] in Fleet Street (Fig. 3). Six of the first seven members of this distinguished group had the Fellowship of the Royal Society and its journal, *Medical Observations and Inquiries*, - published at Fothergill's expense- was said (rather extravagantly) to have 'communicated

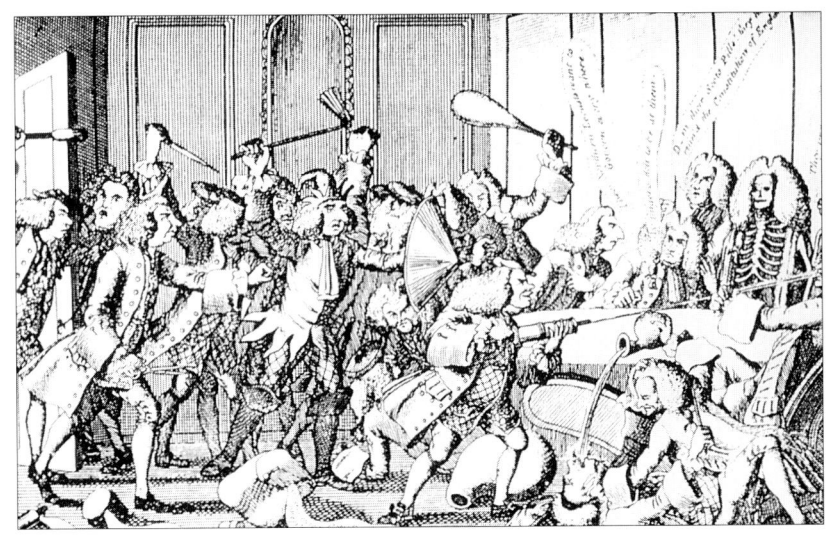

Fig. 2. The invasion of the College of Physicians in Warwick Lane by the Licentiates in 1767.
(By kind permission of the Royal College of Physicians)

to the world more useful information (including, for example, the first account of the pathology of angina of effort) than the College have done in their corporate capacity since the time of their first foundation.' This was clearly a threat which could not be ignored, but when the College started a rival journal, *Medical Transactions*, the Licentiates simply refused to contribute. Yet despite this spirited opposition it was to be another 80 years before the Fellowship of the College was generally available.

John Coakley Lettsom (1744-1815)

The problem of divisions within the ranks of medicine was also tackled by John Coakley Lettsom. Like Fothergill, Lettsom received his training by being carefully channelled through the Quaker community. Starting in Settle as an apprentice to the Yorkshire surgeon/apothecary **Abraham Sutcliffe** he went to London where, with Fothergill's help, he got a job as a dresser at St. Thomas's Hospital. He completed his training at Edinburgh and Leiden and then, having obtained a Licence from the College, started work in London at the age of 26. Lettsom, who was eventually to take over Fothergill's extensive practice, is often presented in a rather unfavourable light. A reputation for social climbing earned him the nick-name Dr. Wriggle and the caption on Rowlandson's cartoon *Physician by his Patient's Deathbed* (I purge, I bleed and sweats 'em, And when they dies I Lets'em) is not exactly complimentary. Moreover, unlike Fothergill, he was reputed always to think first about his fee. This is unfortunate, for although his income was very large, it was earned by hard work and matched by his immense generosity.

Like most of his fellow Quakers he was deeply involved in activities designed to improve the lot of the working class, and his vast

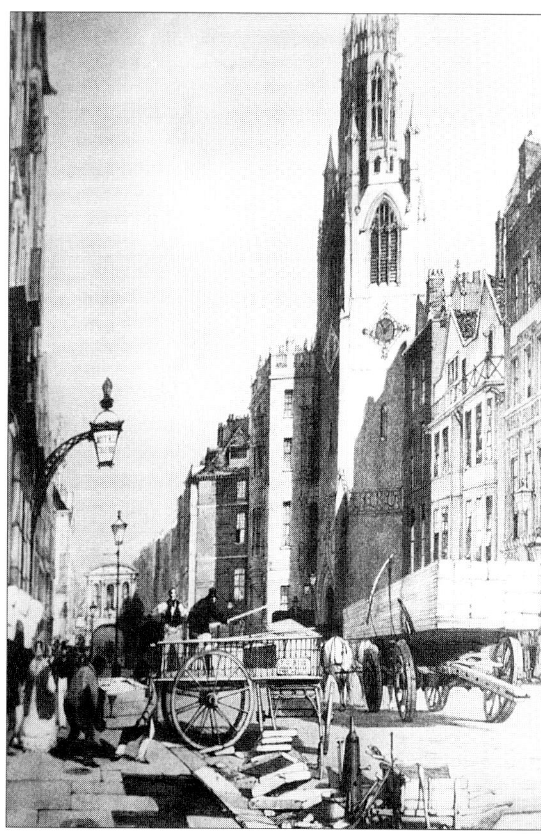

Fig. 3. Fleet Street looking west, with Temple Bar in the distance. The lantern of the Mitre Tavern is on the left, opposite St. Dunstan's church and Crane Court

output of 'reforming' papers included the first account of alcoholism or indeed of any form of drug addiction. He was a friend of Howard, the prison reformer, and at no small risk to himself offered his services to the nearby Wood Street prison. He founded the Royal Sea Bathing Hospital at Margate - the first open air sanatorium - and (following Fothergill's interest in resuscitation) was instrumental in the creation of the Royal Humane Society. But his most significant contributions were the establishment of the dispensary movement and the foundation of the Medical Society of London.

The Dispensary

From their studies of society Quakers had concluded that, given reasonable circumstances, the working class could to a large extent resolve its own problems. The margin of safety was, however, narrow and a period of illness or unemployment quickly upset the fine balance between solvency and distress. Imprisonment for debt, which carried a significant risk of death from gaol fever,[3] was a catastrophe for the entire family. It was therefore essential that, in times of illness or unemployment, the breadwinner - on whose activities both society and his family depended - should immediately receive treatment and/or sufficient support to sustain him and his family until he could return to work. Hitherto during the first half of the eighteenth century, as will be explained in chapter 11, charitable activities had to a large extent been channelled into the provision of civic hospitals. For a minority of (predominantly surgical) patients - and for the medical luminaries that worked in them - such establishments were clearly of considerable value. But for the vast majority of invalids - those with chronic illnesses or fevers, pregnant women and children - they had little to offer. Indeed hospitals were often expressly forbidden to admit such patients. To meet their needs social reformers therefore began to develop an entirely different sort of establishment known as a dispensary.

Like hospitals, dispensaries were staffed by physicians, surgeons and apothecaries. But instead of being admitted to the institution, dispensary patients were seen and treated in a clinic or in their homes. This had four major advantages. There were no constraints on the type of patients who could be seen; there was virtually no limit to the number of patients that could be dealt with; the response was immediate; and the service was a great deal cheaper to run. Unlike hospitals, dispensaries were therefore well able to meet the medical and financial needs of the sick worker. Moreover they proved, on a more general level, to be both informative and useful. The dispensary staff, whose work kept them in close contact with their patients, had an unrivalled knowledge of the living and working conditions of the poor and of the diseases from which they suffered. Dispensaries were therefore used for teaching, and in both Leeds and York the dispensary was an integral part of the medical school. They also served as an invaluable 'early warning station' against the ever-present threat of epidemics, as in Leeds in 1887 when the identification and isolation of thirty-three patients with typhus prevented a major outbreak.

Dispensaries, of course, were not a new invention, for the College of Physicians had attempted to establish one as early as 1687. This was in part the result of a dispute with the apothecaries who, instead of merely dispensing drugs, had started to charge for advice. Despite internal opposition the College therefore decided to retaliate by providing drugs free of charge, and after two abortive attempts a successful service was finally established in 1697. It lasted for thirty years, and was copied by the evangelist John Wesley[4] at Moorfields and Bristol in 1746 and by Armstrong who founded a dispensary for children in 1769. But the movement did not really take shape until 1770, when the twenty-six year old Lettsom (almost certainly aided by Fothergill) founded the dispensary at Aldersgate with Hulme as its first physician. Thereafter the idea spread rapidly, and by the end of the century there were thirteen dispensaries in London alone. It also extended to the provinces, appearing in York and Leeds in 1788 and 1824 respectively.

Curiously, the dispensary system also coincided neatly with the inclinations of the medical staff, many of whom were Quakers trained in Edinburgh. Such men were of course unlikely to obtain prestigious appointments in the hospitals. But Quakers were opposed to the idea of confinement - be it in hospital, asylum or prison - and to the inference of superiority adopted by hospital consultants. It was more in keeping with their beliefs to work on terms of equality with the surgeon and apothecary from the dispensary. Similarly, although the task of the dispensary physician was hard and (because of the risk of infection) potentially dangerous, for men with a strong social conscience it was also very attractive. It was moreover a system within which they could assuage their thirst for knowledge by learning more about diseases and conveying this information to others. The dispensary was therefore an ideal organisation for both the Quaker physician/philanthropist and the working poor.

The Medical Society of London

Closely linked with the dispensary movement was the Medical Society of London. It is usually said that this Society was designed to bring together the three branches of the profession, physicians, surgeons and apothecaries, whose relationships had been soured by commercial disputes and squabbles over social status. In fact, as Booth has pointed out, this may be the very reverse of the truth, for by working on terms of equality in the dispensaries these three groups had already united. But the staff in individual dispensaries, scattered in isolation round the City, had no forum in which they could meet and exchange ideas with their colleagues. The physicians, mainly Licentiates who had graduated in Edinburgh, were not accepted by the College, surgeons without hospital appointments were not accepted at the Surgeons' Hall and apothecaries were not welcome in either. The Society was therefore created to provide the three groups, who had already formed small local units, with a central organisation.

Founded by Lettsom in 1773 and inaugurated under the chairmanship of the first dispensary doctor, Nathaniel Hulme, it was clear from the outset that the Society was no mere dining club. Sometimes known (because of its address) as the Society in Crane Court, it shared with the Royal Society a house off Fleet Street which had once belonged to the son of Thomas Browne. It had both a library and a museum and its academic activities and the widespread reporting of its discussions in its *Memoirs* (which became the voice of the dispensary movement) manifested a characteristically Quaker zeal for knowledge and the dissemination of information. Its journal is in fact the only eighteenth century English medical journal which is still in production. Similarly in 1907, when William Osler persuaded many London medical societies to unite and form the Royal Society of Medicine, the Medical Society of London was one of the few which refused to join - on the grounds that its 'apothecaries' (by now general practitioners) were not adequately represented. It therefore has the additional distinction of being the oldest medical society in the City.

Over the years, the growth of general practice and the increasing cost of medical technology gradually undermined the role of the dispensaries and most have now closed. The buildings, however, often remain. Lacking the architectural splendour of the great civic hospitals of the eighteenth century and the portraits of medical dignitaries that adorn their boardrooms, they are yet a silent reminder of one of the glories of British medicine - of the despised but able physicians, surgeons and apothecaries who, under atrocious circumstances, first brought orthodox treatment to the masses.

REFERENCES

Booth, C.C. Doctors in Science and Society. British Medical Journal 1987.
Booth, C.C. Annual Oration, Medical Society of London. Transactions 1997/98. 114. 79.
Hunt, T. The Medical Society of London. Heinemann 1972.
Kilpatrick, R. 'Living in the Light' - dispensaries, philanthropy and medical reform in late-eighteenth-century London. in Medical Enlightenment in the 18th century. Cunningham, A. Cambridge 1990.
Webb, K.A. 'One of the most useful charities in the city': York Dispensary 1788-1988. University of York Borthwick Papers 74.

NOTES

1. Despite the immense contrast between the splendour of the ecclesiastical hierarchy of Rome and the egalitarian simplicity of the Quakers, the parallels between the two are striking. Both were closely integrated international organisations inspired by Christianity and both laid great store by learning, self-discipline and public service.
2. The Mitre Tavern, now replaced by Hoare's Bank, has many interesting connections. It was the meeting place of the Society of Antiquaries, was frequented by Pepys and Goldsmith and

was reputed to be the place where Boswell first met Johnson. At a later date it was also visited by **Thomas Hodgson**, a Leeds bodysnatcher who lived in a group of cottages in Sheepscar called Resurrection Row. Despite the support of Hey and Thackrah he was jailed repeatedly and in 1833 he moved to Edinburgh where he worked as a porter in the anatomy department. Although, with financial help from his erstwhile customers, he eventually enrolled as a student, he never qualified and when last heard of was working as a bonesetter, doctor and quack lawyer at the Mitre Tavern where he gave consultations from 10.30, seated in Dr. Johnson's old chair.

3. Howard, the prison reformer, died from an infection contracted during a prison visit and Lettsom's only son died of a similar infection caught in the dispensary.
4. Wesley, who 'for six or seven and twenty years made anatomy and physic the diversion of my leisure hours', was acquainted with the works of Boerhaave, Dover, Cheyne and Sydenham but had a poor opinion of doctors because they tended to use numerous technical terms and complicated medicines. His account of the treatments used at his dispensary, published in 1747 under the title of Primitive Physic, was designed to provide the general public with 'a physician always in the house who attends without fee or reward'. Written in the space of three months it was to run through 38 editions, earning the author a substantial amount of money.

CHAPTER IV

Facts and Fevers

*The statistical comparison of results obtained by different doctors
and hospitals is often regarded as a new development.
In fact it is at least three hundred years old.*

ONE OF THE many achievements with which the great post-Revolutionary hospitals of Paris are credited is the introduction of statistical methods into the practice of medicine. Pierre Louis, for example, who taught that 'statistics are the fundamental and only bases of all medical studies', used this technique to discredit the long-established practice of blood-letting. But as is so often the case in medicine, it is not difficult to find earlier examples of others who had done the same thing. There is, for example, a 14th century Arab manuscript which describes a (rather unimpressive) points system for predicting the outcome of an illness. Another more serious contender is John Graunt (1620-74), a London haberdasher. Graunt, who had no medical qualifications, was clearly a person of considerable influence in the City, for at the age of 30 he was able to obtain the Chair of Music at Gresham's College for Sir William Petty, the Oxford anatomist who, on one memorable occasion, helped Willis to revive a recently 'executed' malefactor. More importantly, he had an interest in statistics which he brought to bear on the Bills of Mortality - the records of deaths which, particularly since 1629, parishes had been required to keep. The results of his studies, published in 1662, laid the foundations of what Petty called political arithmetic and so impressed Charles II that he recommended the author as one of the original members of the Royal Society. Indeed he went so far as to advise the Council that 'if they found any more such tradesmen they should be sure to admit them all without more ado' - a perfect example of the egalitarianism that made this upstart society so reprehensible in the eyes of the College of Physicians.

The value of Graunt's studies was clearly appreciated by the Royal Society, for his technique was soon to be applied to another major medical problem. At this time smallpox was still responsible for up to 10% of all deaths. But in 1717 the wife of the British Consul in Constantinople, Lady Mary Wortley Montagu, described to a friend how Turkish women contrived to prevent infection by deliberately inducing mild attacks of the disease, and four years later she had her own daughter 'inoculated' in this way. Those invited to watch the procedure, who included Sir Hans Sloane - President of both the Royal Society and the College of Physicians - were evidently unimpressed. But the experiment did not pass without notice for soon after - when the safety of the technique had been tested on six prisoners from Newgate - the king's grand-daughters were treated in the same way.

Despite this sign of Royal approval inoculation was not generally adopted, for reasons which were set out with remarkable clarity by **William Hillary** (1697-1763) in his book *A rational and mechanical essay on the Small Pox* (1735). Hillary, who at one stage was seeing more than 60 cases a year in his practice in Ripon, pointed out that to make a logical decision about any treatment one had to have a collection of observed facts and the mathematical ability to analyse them. In this instance it had to be shown a) that smallpox induced by inoculation was less dangerous than smallpox caught by infection and b) that it was as effective in preventing a recurrence. In the absence of such data he adopted a conservative approach and, following Boerhaave's advice, continued to recommend bleeding and purging. Hillary seems also to have had an idea that climate might have some bearing on the problem - an idea he first entertained in 1726 but put aside when a **Dr. Wintringham** of York published a similar study, *Commentarium Nosologicum*. In the second edition of his book on smallpox, published in 1740, and in his book on tropical diseases, however, he again considered the effect of climate on 'epidemical' diseases.

In point of fact the information Hillary sought was already available, for the Royal Society had clearly appreciated the importance of Graunt's statistical studies. A survey by James Jurin, Secretary to the Society, revealed that between 1680 and 1722 smallpox had been responsible for one in every fourteen deaths in London, the mortality in severe epidemics reaching 40%. Meantime the Yorkshire physician **Thomas Nettleton** (1683-1742) was comparing the mortality of those who had contracted the disease naturally with that of those who had been inoculated. Together, he and Jurin showed that 'the Small Pox procured by inoculation is far less Dangerous than the same Distemper has been for many Years in the Natural Way'.

These studies were continued by two other statistically-minded physicians who came, once more, from that remarkably fertile area at the head of Wensleydale. **John Haygarth** (1740-1827) was born in Garsdale and, like Fothergill and Willan, was educated at Sedbergh School. Prior to that, however, he had been tutored by an outstanding local physician, **John Dawson** (1734-1820). Dawson, who was also born in Garsdale, began life as a shepherd and contrived to educate himself with the aid of borrowed books. He was then taken on as an assistant to an apothecary in Lancaster, after which he himself worked as an apothecary in Sedbergh. Having earned a little money he walked to Edinburgh, studied medicine for as long as his funds would allow and walked back home again. Two years later he repeated the process, this time journeying to London where he obtained some sort of diploma.

Despite this remarkable background, however, it is not on his training and practice as a physician that Dawson's reputation depends. Rather he is remembered as a mathematician and tutor whose ability, even disregarding his lack of formal education, was phenomenal. It was he, for example, who challenged the Professor of Mathematics at Edinburgh University, correctly insisting that the only way to calculate the distance between the earth and the sun was to observe the transit of the planet Venus - an exercise which was carried out by another Yorkshireman, **James Cook**, on his first great voyage. Among Dawson's distinguished pupils were Robert Willan, Adam Sedgwick the famous geologist, a future headmaster of Harrow and no fewer than 12 senior wranglers. For present purposes, however, it is with the assistance he gave to Haygarth in the mathematical analysis of his observations that we are concerned.

Haygarth spent most of his life at Chester or in Bath. Like many contemporary physicians he was greatly influenced by the work of Sydenham and by his studies of epidemic fevers. He was, however, unable to accept Sydenham's argument that they were in some way caused by the constitution of the patient and the nature of the air. After studying cases of smallpox and analysing Bills of Mortality he came to the conclusion that, at least in this instance, infection was caused by close contact with a person suffering from the disease. Airborne spread was possible, but only at a distance of a few feet. He published his findings in *An Inquiry into how to Prevent the Small Pox* (1784), incorporating Dawson's calculations of the probability of one or more individuals in a group of people exposed to the disease escaping infection, assuming that a certain proportion of the community was immune. He also calculated the extent to which the population would increase were the disease to be eradicated.

Eradication, thanks to Haygarth's efforts, was more than a hypothetical idea, for as early as 1778 he had established a Smallpox Society in Chester and was discussing a plan for the elimination of the disease in the U.K. with Fothergill. In part this scheme was based on a policy of regular and widespread inoculation. But Haygarth, like Petty (who edited the later editions of Graunt's books) also realised the importance of keeping victims away from the healthy population. This was not an entirely new idea, for in his book *Utopia* (1516) Sir Thomas More envisaged for his perfect city hospitals with wards 'so big, so wide, so ample that they which were taken and holden with contagious diseases such as would by infection to crape from one to another might be laid apart.' Haygarth took this idea to its logical conclusion when, in 1783, he introduced the first isolation wards for patients with fevers at Chester Hospital. In 1793 his policies were brought together in a *Sketch of a plan to exterminate the casual smallpox from Great Britain and to introduce General Inoculation*. Based on this combination of inoculation and isolation, it specified clearly rewards and punishments designed to ensure the co-operation of the public. It was of course to be another 200 years before the World Health Organisation, by implementing what were essentially Haygarth's ideas, finally contrived to eradicate the disease. But Haygarth did live to see the introduction of vaccination[1] in 1796 and it was he who provided Professor Waterhouse of Harvard with material to carry out the first vaccination in America in 1800 - on his own children, one of whom was subsequently (and uneventfully) inoculated with smallpox to test the efficacy of the procedure.

The study of infectious diseases was to be continued in Wensleydale during the twentieth century. During the Second World War a distinguished American epidemiologist expressed a wish to meet a colleague working in the same field. Told by the Ministry of Health that he would be brought to London he replied 'No sir! I want to meet him in that goddam little country town where he does his work.' So it was that John Gordon, Professor of Epidemiology at Harvard University met **William Pickles** (1889-1969), general practitioner at Aysgarth. The meeting went well, although Pickles was ashamed to show his guest a sanatorium full of children with (bovine)[2] tuberculous adenitis or osteomyelitis - conditions which the American had not previously encountered - and in due course the Yorkshire G.P was to add the Cutter Lecture at Harvard to an ever-growing list of honours.

Pickles, who was to become one of the most famous general practitioners of the twentieth century and the first president of the Royal College of General Practitioners, had trained at Leeds. Despite being Moynihan's dresser, his early academic career was anything but distinguished. He went into practice at Aysgarth, but it was not until he was 41 that, having read the biographies of men like Jenner and Mackenzie, he realised the potential value of clinical observations made in general practice. His decision to study epidemic fevers may have been prompted by an outbreak of typhoid he had encountered in Bedale some years earlier. On that occasion, correctly surmising that the problem was caused by a gypsy woman washing her ailing husband's clothes at the village pump, he used the technique Snow had used to end the cholera epidemic in Soho and curtailed the outbreak by putting the pump out of action.

The work which was to make him famous was, however, far less dramatic for, as he modestly explained, 'it concerned very simple things, everyday happenings and elementary deductions drawn from them'. He had become interested in the spread of infectious diseases through the scattered communities in his area - first of infectious hepatitis and then of Bornholm disease and Sonne dysentery. This led to a prolonged survey the basis of which was indeed very simple. For each of the communities round Aysgarth, Pickles (or rather his wife) prepared a calendar/chart. Using different symbols for each disease, he entered on these charts the day of onset of the various infectious fevers he encountered. By studying the movement of people between these remote communities he then tried to work out the shortest time between an isolated 'contact' and the onset of symptoms. In this way he was able to establish the incubation period of the various disorders.

The work was presented at the Royal Society of Medicine in 1935 and was hailed as 'the most outstanding contribution to epidemiology for twenty-five years.' Like many other famous manuscripts, however, it was rejected by several of the leading publishers. But when it eventually appeared in 1939 *Epidemiology in a Country Practice* rapidly became a medical classic. As Pickles observed (quoting Sir Thomas Browne) 'I do not secretly implore and wish for great plagues'; but, he added, 'the presence of a little infectious disease is not without its thrill.'

REFERENCES
Booth, C.C. Doctors in Science and Society. British Medical Journal 1987.
Pemberton, J. Will Pickles of Wensleydale. London, Bles, 1970.

NOTES
1. Vaccination is the prevention of smallpox by inducing an infection with the closely related cowpox virus. This was less dangerous than the existing technique of inoculation (variolation), in which the objective was to induce a mild attack of smallpox itself.
2. A form of tuberculosis contracted from the milk of infected cattle.

CHAPTER V

Medical Artists

In many medical publications the provision of good illustrations is of crucial importance. Yorkshire has interesting links with two men who did such work.

IN THE LAST analysis, the success of a textbook of anatomy depends on the skill of the artist employed to do the illustrations. It is therefore remarkable that the name of this important individual is so often forgotten. Vesalius' *de Humani Corporis Fabrica*, for example, is one of the most famous books ever published, and Vesalius deserves great credit both for his skill as an anatomist and for his determination to use the best artist and printer available. But the book, which has been said to be 'more admired and less read than any other publication of equal significance in the history of medicine', is treasured for its illustrations and not for its text. Yet despite much speculation, the name of the artist who produced them remains unknown.

Nearer to us in time and place the same could be said of Gray's Anatomy. First published in 1858, it is perhaps the best known of all medical texts. Yet the man who drew the illustrations which are the very essence of the book remains virtually unknown. He was in fact **Henry Vandyke Carter** (1831-1897), who came from and is buried at Scarborough. The son of a local water-colour painter, he was educated at University College, St. George's Hospital and the Charite Hospital in Paris. When he had qualified his father wanted him to return to Scarborough as assistant to a local physician but Carter, aware of his potential, rejected this idea with the comment that he was 'fit for a higher office.' Realising the commercial value of the artistic skills he had inherited he placed an advertisement in the Lancet of March 19th 1853 which read 'A young gentleman M.R.C.S. and acquainted with pathology, the microscope etc., is desirous of assisting Gentlemen engaged in scientific research by making drawings.' It was an advertisement which should have established his name, for it led to his most fruitful partnership with Henry Gray of St. George's Hospital. But whereas Gray's name is indelibly stamped on the face of medicine Carter lapsed into obscurity, joining the Indian Medical Service where he became Professor of Anatomy at Bombay and, among other things, gave the first description of relapsing fever in India.

There seems in fact to be only one group of medical artists who can be assured of full recognition - those who draw their own anatomical dissections. Examples include Leonardo, whose illustrations - unpublished until they were discovered in the Royal Archives at Windsor nearly four centuries later - are perhaps even better than those of Vesalius, and Charles Bell. The thirty plates in Bell's System of Dissection, written while he was yet a student, are said to be among the finest ever published, and his engravings of the brain which appeared four years later have been equated with those of Vesalius and Willis. But Yorkshire can also boast a distinguished artist/anatomist whose early efforts in this field brought him into contact with one of the most picturesque medical men the county has produced.

John Burton (1701-1771) was a well-known figure in York society, for besides being a leading obstetrician and one of the founding physicians of the York hospital he was an eminent antiquarian. He was also a man whose political activities and outbursts of violence had made him many enemies. In 1745 these problems came home to roost.

Following his victory at Prestonpans in the 'forty-five' rebellion Charles Stuart, the Young Pretender, had started to march south. He had reached Kendal and would in due course get as far as Derby, but at this stage nobody knew whether he would advance through Lancashire or through York. To Dr. Burton this was a matter of great concern, for even if York was spared he had properties in Lancashire from which he wished to collect the rents. After discussing his problem with the Recorder he therefore hurried inland to Settle and, having concluded his business, went on to an inn at Hornby to stay the night. There he was found by a group of Scots horsemen who took him to Lancaster for questioning. He was released almost at once, but not before news of his capture had been conveyed to York where political enemies, led by the Precentor, Dr. Jacques Sterne, created the impression that he was a Jacobite and a Papist whose meeting with the Scots had been pre-arranged. A warrant was issued for his arrest - signed, among others, by Dr. Sterne - bail was refused and he was incarcerated in York Castle. There further accusations, almost certainly engineered, led to a charge of treason and three months later, despite being crippled with gout, he was taken to London for questioning by the Privy Council. He was, in fact, in a very precarious position, for in York and elsewhere large numbers of 'rebels' were being executed. In this respect Burton was fortunate as he was only detained for 16 months, during which time he exercised his antiquarian interests by cataloguing the charters, patents and escheat rolls in the Tower of London. But his imprisonment cost him £700, his investments and his position as senior physician at the York County Hospital. It was therefore hardly surprising that, when he was eventually released without prosecution, this pugnacious individual should publish a pamphlet entitled *British Liberty Endangered*.

This, however, was not Burton's only problem. His main interest in medicine was obstetrics - he had, among other things, invented some rather unsatisfactory obstetric forceps - and he was writing a treatise on the subject. But he now found that 'a person' (the obstetrician Dr. Smellie) 'was going to publish my improvements with some work of his own'. It therefore became a matter of urgency to get his book, and in particular the illustrations for his book, prepared as rapidly as possible. And here his fortune changed when he met George Stubbs.

George Stubbs (1724-1806) was the son of a Liverpool leather dresser. From an early age it was known that he had considerable artistic ability and he was twice sent for professional training - in England and to Rome which, at the time, was the Mecca of the artistic world. Both episodes were, however, brief and in the event he was self-taught, preferring, as he said (in words reminiscent of Boyle's instructions to scientists) 'to look into nature for himself and consult and study her alone.' He clearly had a particular interest in natural history, for in childhood he started to draw bones and anatomical dissections loaned to him by a local doctor and in his teens he dissected and drew dogs and horses in his father's shop. This, however, was not his only talent, for on leaving home he first went to Leeds where for a short time he painted portraits. In 1745 he moved on to York, and it was there that his interest in anatomy became known to a local surgeon, Mr. Charles Atkinson, who began to supply him with human bodies for dissection. So successful were his activities in this field that within a short time he was giving lectures in anatomy and becoming more than a little involved in the body-snatching escapades required to sustain his interest. Indeed it was probably because of these activities that he was held 'in vile regard' in the locality.

If Stubbs was unpopular with the citizens of York, to Dr. Burton, now once more at liberty, the discovery of someone who was both artist and anatomist was a godsend, for he was ideally qualified to do the illustrations for his book. With that end in mind the body of a pregnant woman was stolen and brought to Stubbs' house for dissection. The necessary drawings were soon done but difficulties arose over the engravings, for local craftsmen were unwilling to handle such distasteful material. Stubbs overcame this problem by returning to Leeds, consulting an acquaintance who had some experience of this sort of work and learning enough about the process to engrave the 18 plates himself.

Burton's *Essay Towards a Complete New System of Midwifery* was published in 1751. It was not an unqualified success. The artist himself refused to have his name associated with the book, for he was far from satisfied with the engravings (Fig.4). They were indeed inferior to the magnificent illustrations drawn by Jan van Rymsdyk for William Hunter's *Anatomy of the Human Gravid Uterus*, but those pictures were based on three or four hundred dissections - all of which must have been done on stolen bodies, for it was illegal to hang a pregnant woman. As far as the profession was concerned it took little notice of the book, preferring the work by Dr. Smellie - a slight which moved Burton, with all the tact that had created political enemies, to publish *'A letter to William Smellie M.D. containing critical and practical remarks upon his treatise on the Theory and Practice of Midwifery wherein gross mistakes and dangerous methods of practice recommended by the author are fully demonstrated and generally corrected.'* Finally, to add insult to injury, Laurence Sterne, Vicar of the nearby village of Coxwold and

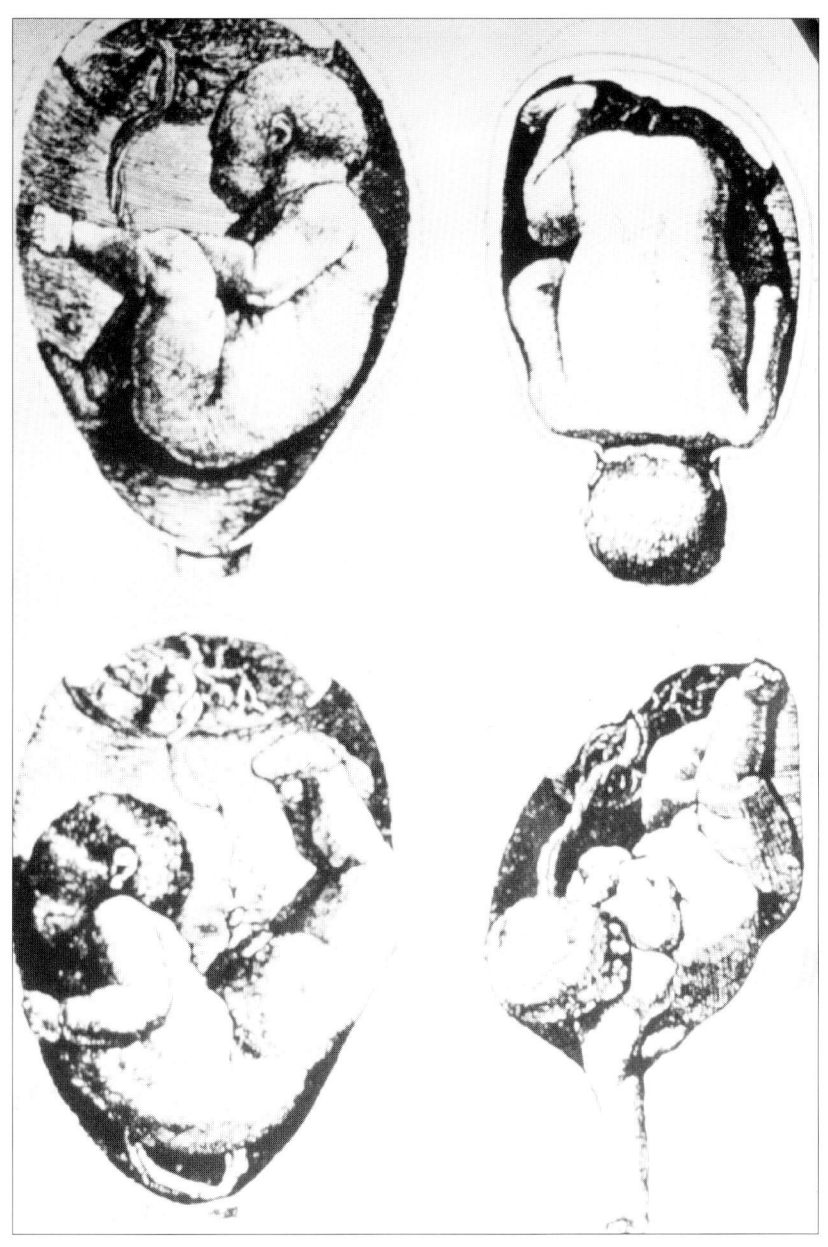

Fig. 4. Engravings prepared by George Stubbs for John Burton's treatise on obstetrics.

nephew of Burton's old enemy at the Minster, caricatured him and his obstetric forceps in the grotesque figure of Dr. Slop in *Tristram Shandy*.[1]

Stubbs' career, by contrast, continued to develop. By degrees he began to concentrate on painting horses and other animals, a skill which was in great demand at a time when country houses and country pursuits were much in vogue. This had the unfortunate effect of overshadowing his ability in the more highly esteemed field of portrait painting, and although in due course he was offered an R.A. it was never conferred. Indeed until the beginning of the 20th century, when he was hailed as one of the greatest painters the country has ever produced, his name was virtually forgotten. But nothing could conceal the genius of his masterpiece, his book on equine anatomy. This amazing work was based on studies which began in 1758 in a remote farmhouse near the village of Horkstow on the south bank of the Humber. He probably chose this secluded place because his interest in anatomy had attracted unwelcome attention at York and because of the revolting nature of the work he was about to undertake. This involved the killing (by bleeding) of a great many horses whose vessels were then injected with tallow before they were hauled up and posed in a standing position. They were then dissected, layer by layer, down to the skeleton - a process which took six or seven (and in one case eleven) weeks. The physical task of positioning these large animals - with which he had only the help of his mistress - was immense. The olfactory horrors of working indoors with an unpreserved corpse for a period of two or three months defy description.

After spending 18 months on the preparation of his illustrations Stubbs went to London in search of an engraver. Once more, however, because such studies were still viewed with suspicion, he was unable to find anyone willing to undertake the task. Over the next six years he therefore set about preparing the 24 engravings himself, working on commissions during the day and on his anatomical plates at night. His book, *The Anatomy of the Horse*, was eventually published in 1766 and was immediately hailed by both artists and anatomists as a work of genius, earning Stubbs a place among the greatest natural scientists England has produced and alongside Leonardo as a scientific artist.

York has no memorial to Stubbs. Burton's memorial in Holy Trinity, Micklegate, takes the form of a charter supported by two books - the great antiquarian survey *Monasticon Eboracense* to which he devoted much of his life (Fig. 5). But medical historians might feel that there should also be a third, smaller book to commemorate the links between a distinguished Yorkshire obstetrician, a famous Yorkshire novelist and the first attempt at anatomical engravings by one of England's leading artists.

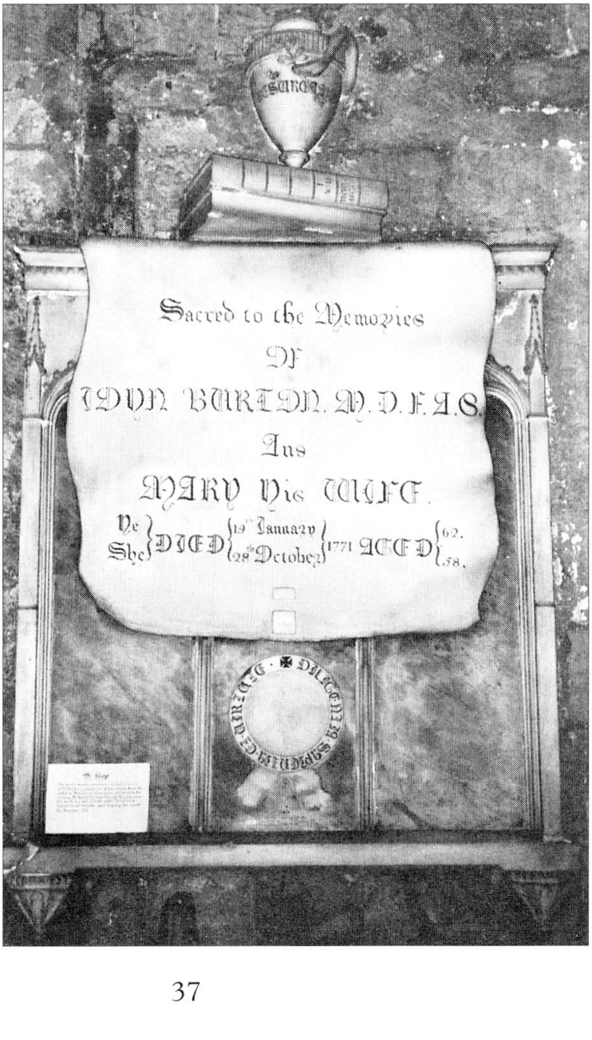

Fig. 5. John Burton's memorial in Holy Trinity, Micklegate, York showing the two volumes of his Monasticon Eboracense.

REFERENCES

Bayliss, A.M. Dr. Henry Vandyke Carter (1831-1897). Yorkshire History Quarterly 1998. Vol.4 No.2. 69.

Fountain, R.B. George Stubbs as an Anatomist. Proceedings of the Royal Society of Medicine 1968. 61. 639.

Parker, C.A. Mr. Stubbs the Horse Painter. Allen 1971.

Davies, R. Memoirs of Richard Burton, M.D., F.S.A. Yorkshire Archaeological Journal 1873. 2.403.

NOTES

1. It was some small compensation that in due course Sterne's own body was 'snatched' by resurrectionists, subsequently appearing on a slab in the department of anatomy at Cambridge. Here the sight of it so alarmed the friend who recognised it that he fainted with shock. This, however, did not interrupt the proceedings, for when his remains were recovered 200 years later during the clearing of a burial ground on the Bayswater Road the vault of the skull had been removed. After comparing the (unusually small) measurements of the vault with those of a bust by Nollekens, Sterne's remains were reburied in his churchyard at Coxwold.

CHAPTER VI

Psychiatry

For many years the 'care' of the insane consisted of a mixture of confinement and restraint. Yorkshire played a major part in the development of more humane methods in what were to be the first hospitals devoted to one medical specialty.

BY THE 18th CENTURY it had become evident that the established methods of medical treatment - bleeding, cupping, purging etc - were at best useless, and patients and doctors alike began to experiment with new techniques such as hydrotherapy,[1] mesmerism and galvanism. Some of these methods, like the magnetic tractors patented by Elisha Perkins of Connecticut, were every bit as ridiculous as those they sought to replace. This divider-like contraption, made of various metals, was supposed, on stroking the skin, to have the effect of galvanism - an idea richly satirised in cartoons such as one headed 'A Terrible Tractoration'. But the technique was not finally discredited until **John Haygarth**, who by now had moved to Bath, showed in his paper *'On the imagination as a cause and a cure of disorders of the body'* (1800) that similar 'cures' could be effected with a device made of wood.

This article by a Yorkshire physician would be of little interest were it not for a second paper on an almost identical subject read nearly a century later. In 1869 the British Medical Association, no doubt attracted by the opening of the revolutionary new Infirmary, held its annual meeting in Leeds. Among the visitors was the eminent French physician Jean-Martin Charcot, who was to hear a paper by Russell Reynolds on *'Paralysis and other disorders of motion and sensation dependent on idea'* (ie on what is now known as hysteria). This presentation was to have a major effect on Charcot's future activities. Hitherto his main interest had been in organic diseases of the nervous system, but during the course of a reorganisation of his own hospital he had just taken over the care of such psychiatric patients in the Salpetriere as were not deemed to be mad. They came, moreover, with an 'alienist' (psychiatrist) called Bourneville who already had an interest in hysteria. As a result of these events Charcot's own studies turned increasingly in this direction and, perhaps unfortunately, he is now remembered more for his spectacular demonstrations of hysterical patients than for his seminal work in the field of organic neurology. More important still, he had among his followers at that time a young Austrian student, Sigmund Freud, who was translating Charcot's famous lectures into German. Directly and indirectly, therefore, Russell Reynolds' Leeds' paper - to which Charcot frequently referred - had a major influence on the development of psychiatry.

The York Lunatic Asylum

Psychiatry was certainly in need of development, for although the trial and execution of 'witches' (like that in which Thomas Browne participated) had ceased, the standard response to insanity was incarceration. In France huge 'hospitals', often under ecclesiastical control, were used as a dumping ground for the mad, the bad, the poor, the aged, the disabled, orphans, prostitutes and other 'undesirables'. England, which had lost its monasteries in the Dissolution,[2] had no comparable facilities and those who were deemed to be mad had to be detained on a piecemeal basis. Some, like a man admitted to the West Riding Lunatic Asylum in 1823, were simply confined by the family. This particular patient had been shut in a cupboard under the stairs for eleven years, with the result that he had lost the ability to stand. Some were left in the care of a custodian appointed by the parish. Some, found wandering away from home, were committed to prison and may even have been executed. But the majority were confined in the local workhouse which often had an area set aside for 'pauper lunatics and idiots'.

For the more opulent there was, however, the alternative of a private madhouse - the basis of the lucrative 'trade in lunacy'. These institutions varied considerably in the facilities they offered. At one extreme, as at Ticehurst House in Sussex, inmates had their own houses and cooks and were able to go out hunting. For the majority, however, the prospect was far less attractive. Prior to the 1774 Act for the Regulation of Private Mad Houses patients admitted by relatives had virtually no means of escape and even after that it was clearly not in the financial interests of the proprietor that they should recover. It was therefore hardly surprising that at the start of the 19th century there were 5,000 patients in such establishments and a further 5,000 in workhouses.

The predicament of these patients, who were often detained without treatment under atrocious conditions, attracted the attention of the 18th century philanthropists. Yorkshire in particular saw the development of three institutions that were to play a major part in improving their circumstances, developing new methods of treatment and - as was often the case with large asylums - promoting an understanding of the structure and function of the brain. This movement started in York in 1772 when a group of citizens, which included William Wilberforce, MP for Yorkshire, 'sensible of the deplorable situation of poor lunaticks in this extensive county who have no support but what a needy parent can bestow or a thrifty parish officer provide' resolved to follow four other cities and 'subscribe towards a public edifice for the reception of these unhappy people'. The design of the building was left in the hands of John Carr, architect of the original Infirmary at Leeds and of Harewood House, and the elegant York Lunatic Asylum (now Bootham Park Hospital) was opened in 1777. Incredibly the 30 or so beds - soon to be doubled in number - were designed to serve the entire county.

The first forty years were a disaster. In large measure this stemmed from a decision to cater, not only for paupers but also for 'persons of moderate circumstances who .... have no place to retire to but a private mad house where their cure stands a great chance of being protracted for the benefit of a mercenary keeper'. Worse still, in addition to being paid a salary, the sole medical officer evidently contrived to charge his more affluent patients. The predictable consequences of this policy only came to light in 1790 following the death of a Quaker patient. Critics pointed out that whereas the original intention had been to provide an asylum for 'the poor and the poor only' the 'defrauded public' had in fact contrived to finance 'a palace for the opulent lunatic' in which 'money from affluent patients was viewed as private profit'.

Following this crisis the Quaker community, led by the Tukes, established its own asylum, the Retreat at York, of which more will be said later. Meanwhile the York Lunatic Asylum continued as before, the unwary Governors accepting a homely boardroom, an obsequious staff and optimistic reports as evidence that all was well. They would indeed have ignored a second case of ill-treatment of a pauper patient in 1813 had not a group of interested citizens, egged on by the Tukes, recalled that on payment of £20 one could become a governor. Gaining access to the administration in this way they were enabled to conduct a thorough investigation of the institution, which revealed a lamentable state of affairs.

Conditions for the affluent patients were found to be satisfactory but elsewhere, as one investigator reported, 'being pretty well acquainted with the receptacles for the poor, with prisons, workhouses and hospitals, I can unhesitatingly assert that I never met with anything approaching the filthy and wretched state of the inferior parts of the asylum' where '100 poor creatures were shut up together unattended and uninspected'. Attendants were in short supply, for there were only seven keepers for 199 inmates, whereas the Retreat had one for every ten. Worse still, it was discovered that nearly a third of the 341 deaths known to have occurred had gone unreported and (when the steward inadvertently submitted two different sets of accounts for the same period) it transpired that the physician was pocketing substantial sums of money to which he was not entitled. These revelations precipitated long-overdue reforms, after which conditions improved considerably. Indeed by 1909 two visiting American doctors reported that it was 'the most progressive institution they had visited in Europe.'

Pinel's theories and the Retreat

The treatment of insanity during the eighteenth and early nineteenth centuries left much to be desired, for the main weapons were sequestration and restraint. In part, as in the case of the Barnsley woman chained to a workhouse wall for 36 years, this was simply designed to take the patient out of circulation. But it was also supposed to 'maximise the prospect of recovery by imposing a sense of calm'. To this end various devices including straps, handcuffs, steel waistcoats, straight-jackets and darkened cells were widely used at least up to the middle of the 19th century. As a secondary measure, steps were taken to 'deplete the frenzied constitution and calm the mind, thus rendering it receptive to reason'. So it was that in 1804 the retiring physician in York 'imparted the mysteries of this obscure branch of medicine' to his successor and taught him how to mix green and grey insane powder (a purgative and an emetic). To this were added opiates, alcohol, mustard plasters, cold douches, leeches, cupping and above all bleeding, as a result of which many of those admitted were in a 'quite appalling state, having been bled almost to death'. Most feared of all was the rotating chair, occasionally used at Wakefield until about 1820, the mere mention of which would often pacify a difficult patient. To Charles Dickens (1852) it seemed that 'Coercion of the outward man and rabid physicking the inward man ..... were the specifics of lunacy. Chains, straw, filthy solitude, darkness and starvation: jalap, syrup of buckthorn, tartarised antimony and ipecacuanha .... in fabulous doses to every patient, whether well or ill. Spinning in whirligigs, corporal punishment, gagging, 'continued intoxication' - nothing was too wildly extravagant, nothing too monstrously cruel to be prescribed by mad doctors'.

In point of fact there was, by this time, a strong reaction against this policy of restraint and 'depletion'. In 1806 **Daniel Davis** (a Sheffield obstetrician who was present at the birth of Queen Victoria) produced an English translation of Pinel's *Treatise on Insanity*. Pinel, whose statue stands outside the Salpetriere in Paris, was renowned for removing the chains from the patients in the Bicetre asylum, and by degrees his approach to mental illness came to be accepted in the United Kingdom. The objective of this new form of treatment was to keep the patient under control with physical activity and to try, by working on the residual normal emotions, to ease the mind back into its correct channels. As Crichton-Browne (1872) explained 'the moral atmosphere of the house, its quiet routines, lessons of gentleness and forbearance, the sway of the sound and strong mind over the diseased and feeble one .... a few kind and well chosen words, a little judicious firmness, a hope suggested, a fear allayed or a new line of thought pointed out is sometimes as beneficial as poppy and mandrake'. So, by the end of the 19th century, even attacks of acute mania were being treated with great success without resorting to opiates.

Among the first establishments to adopt this new approach was the Retreat at York. The opening of this hospital was precipitated by the death of Hannah Mills in the Asylum. As already mentioned, this Quaker patient had been admitted on March 15th 1790 and died on April 29th 1790 before any Quakers were allowed to see her or to offer her religious comfort. This episode came to the notice of **William Tuke**[3] (1732-1822), a Quaker tea merchant of York who had little faith in the medical profession and indeed wondered if they should be allowed to care for the insane. In 1796 he responded by founding an establishment which 'aimed to create a domestic environment to avoid brutalisation' and to replace drugs with 'mildness, reason and community support'. Originally for Quakers only, the Retreat subsequently opened its doors to all denominations.

In spite of this new venture Tuke, his son Henry and his grandson Samuel continued to take an interest in the York Lunatic Asylum and were in large measure responsible for the reform of that establishment. **Samuel Tuke's** (1784-1857) *Description of the Retreat* was however bitterly resented by the staff of the Asylum as it pointed out that medical treatment was useless and extolled the virtues of 'moral' therapy. This posed a commercial threat, for this 'milder' treatment was also used in the private asylum run by the medical director of the Retreat. Samuel Tuke - whose advice was widely sought on such matters - must also have offended the founders of the elegant Asylum at York when he congratulated the magistrates of West Yorkshire on 'preferring internal convenience to external decoration and the comfort of the inmates to the gratification of the passing traveller' in the design of the County Asylum. Nor was he the only member of his family to criticise such waste, for **Daniel Hack Tuke** (1827-95) thought that the new asylum at Meanwood, Leeds 'may very possibly one day be utilised as an asylum for the middle and upper classes' (!) and that it 'would have been wise to avoid .... costly embellishments calculated to prejudice the minds of the ratepayers on entering the building'. By now the Tukes were able to provide a professional as well as a social opinion, for Daniel Tuke had studied medicine on the Continent and published a prize essay on the reformation of treatment since Pinel's work and a well respected manual of psychiatry. He also taught at York Medical School where, among the students he took to the Retreat, was Hughlings Jackson.

The West Riding Lunatic Asylum (Stanley Royd Hospital)

In the first half of the 19th century the task of providing accommodation for psychiatric patients gradually passed from private into public hands. In 1808 county councils were merely empowered to raise funds for mental hospitals but by 1845 they were required so to do. By 1870 (a century after the York Lunatic Asylum opened its 30 beds) Yorkshire had five borough or county hospitals and two registered hospitals. Such institutions - the first hospitals to be set aside for one medical speciality - played a major part in the observation and classification of psychiatric disorders.

The West Riding decided to avail itself of the right to raise funds for an asylum in 1815 - the sixth county to adopt this policy. Initially there was some doubt as to how many beds would be required, for when they first heard of the project parish officers offered every patient who might conceivably have been acceptable. This enthusiasm quickly waned, however, when they were informed of the cost, and in the event the difficulty was one of getting patients referred in the early stages of their illness. The number of beds to be provided was eventually fixed at 150, partly because, in the opinion of the medical superintendent, 'beyond that number patients cease to excite the interest they ought'. Little did he know that by 1908 there would be 2,000 beds and by 1935, 2,500!

The building, which was set on the outskirts of Wakefield, was designed - on the advice of Samuel Tuke - to be humane and functional rather than elegant. To this end it had separate bedrooms for most of the patients and glass instead of bars on the windows. On the other hand it was so planned that everyone - staff as well as patients - could be kept under observation, 'education and talent being but an imperfect security against the seductions of interest and indolence'. It also incorporated an ingenious system for heating and ventilation which, sadly, proved to be a failure.

The most striking feature of the new asylum, however, was the regime which evolved under a succession of talented directors who included, for a brief period, the illustrious **Henry Maudsley** (1835-1918) who was born in Settle. Central to this was the occupation of the patients' time, not only with work (for they were responsible for all the cooking, cleaning, laundry-work, farming etc) but also with entertainments. These were conducted on a grand scale with concerts, plays (in which W S Gilbert once participated), balls, fancy dress parties, fetes, galas, picnics at Walton

Hall (home of Squire Waterton - see p76) and trips to the asylum's own hotel at Redcar. These activities attracted considerable interest in the locality, the citizens of Wakefield coming to watch or to participate in various scientific and social events. Such activities, coupled with an enlightened approach to treatment, rapidly enhanced the reputation of the Asylum which, by 1844, was considered to be among the three best in the country. Its place in history, however, depends mainly on its contribution to neuroscientific research which will be considered in the next chapter.

REFERENCES
Ashworth, A.L. Stanley Royd Hospital, Wakefield.
Digby, A. From York Lunatic Asylum to Bootham Park Hospital. York University Borthwick Papers No. 69.
Goetz, C.G., Bonduelle, M. and Gelfand, T. Charcot. Oxford 1995 p. 178.
Roberts, J. Madhouse to Modecate - Psychiatry in West Yorkshire, 1750-1986. University of Leeds Review 1987/8.30.164.

NOTES
1. It was at this time that the main development of the great spa at Harrogate took place although it, and the much smaller and less well known Gipton Spa in Gledhow Woods, Leeds, were first used in the seventeenth century.
2. One of which, at Barking, specialised in the care of the 'Barking mad'.
3. The Tuke family also manufactured cocoa and chocolate in their shop in Castlegate - a business which was transferred to the Rowntrees in 1862.

CHAPTER VII

'A Scientific Phrenology'

One of Yorkshire's most important contributions to medicine was the confirmation, at the West Riding Lunatic Asylum (Stanley Royd Hospital), that certain parts of the brain are associated with certain functions. It was this discovery that made neurosurgery possible.

JAMES CRICHTON BROWNE (1840-1938), one of the early directors of the West Riding Lunatic Asylum, was a well known figure in Victorian society. A popular speaker, his lofty frame, elegant dress and flowing side-whiskers made him a perfect subject for a Spy cartoon (back cover). But he was also a man of vision and drive who established a most enlightened regime in the institution he governed, publicised its scientific facilities and attracted leading neurologists and psychiatrists to work and speak there. He was the first asylum director to appoint a resident pathologist and it was from this laboratory that the description of the Bevan Lewis cells in the motor cortex emanated. Even more remarkable, however, was the way in which he managed to interest the local population, which already attended concerts and dances at the asylum, in his scientific 'Conversaziones.' Held in the hall - a vast room heated by six huge open fires - it was here that some of the most important physiological studies of that era were first presented. Accounts of these meetings were subsequently published in the *Reports of the West Riding Lunatic Asylum* whose six volumes were the direct predecessor of the journal *Brain*. Indeed, among the first four editors of *Brain* were three of the editors of the Reports - Crichton Browne himself and his colleagues Hughlings Jackson and David Ferrier. It is with the work of the last two that this chapter is mainly concerned.

The origins of cerebral localisation

To appreciate the work of this group - Yorkshire's greatest contribution to scientific neurology - one has to know something of contemporary ideas about the function of the brain. Well into the second half of the nineteenth century the cerebral hemispheres were regarded, not as a collection of 'nerve centres' which subserved movement, sensation, speech, sight etc, but as a unified structure that represented the mind. It had been observed that lesions in one hemisphere tended to produce weakness on the opposite side of the body, but pigeons and other animals from which the hemispheres had been removed seemed to be able to move. Moreover, various attempts to stimulate the cortex electrically or mechanically (including one study on a recently executed prisoner from Newgate) had been unsuccessful. On the other hand stimulation of the lower part of the brain, the medulla, produced violent movements. In his standard textbook of 1878 Wilks therefore concluded that 'it has not been clearly proved that a lesion of a convolution (ie of the cortex of the hemispheres) will produce paralysis of any part of the body. True paralysis is associated with disease of the spinal cord.' In other words, the great mass of the brain was a single organ that governed 'the mind' and other higher functions. More fundamental things like movement were controlled by the brain stem and the cord.

Sadly, the one man who came close to the truth followed an attractive but false line of thought. Franz Joseph Gall (1758-1828) was a distinguished neuro-anatomist who, with Spurzheim, had contrived to demonstrate the decussation of the great motor (pyramidal) tracts - no mean feat at a time when brains could not be hardened prior to examination. Gall had also observed impairment of speech following a sword wound in the frontal lobes. Unfortunately, having noticed that people with a good visual memory tended to have prominent eyes, he concluded that this was due to over-development of the frontal lobes (ie the area concerned with speech) with consequent compression of the orbits. From this he went on to argue that other parts of the cortex with special functions might also hypertrophy and produce prominence of the other parts of the skull. This led to the 'science' of phrenology - informed palpation of the skull to detect such areas of hypertrophy and their associated talents.

This was an attractive idea and one which appealed to many people, including Crichton Browne himself. Sadly it was also counter-productive, for it drew attention away from the crucial underlying observation that certain parts of the cerebral hemisphere have a specific function. Consequently, when phrenology was discredited the idea of cerebral localisation was abandoned at the same time. From other quarters, however, evidence continued to accumulate. The speech centre, first discovered by an obscure French general practitioner some twenty-five years earlier, was re-described by Broca and Todd showed that lesions of the cortex (mostly cerebral tuberculomas) could cause focal fits in children. Experimental studies were also proving to be more rewarding. Fritsch and Hitzig, who had noticed twitching movements in the limbs during the dressing of head wounds, had produced some jerks in response to cortical stimulation and some weakness after ablation of part of the cortex. But the most remarkable experiments of all were conducted by Robert Bartholow, Professor of Medicine at Ohio. Bartholow had a feeble-minded maid who had a cranial epithelioma which had exposed part of the brain. By repeatedly inserting needles into her brain and delivering electric shocks he contrived in turn to produce focal tingling, focal jerking and full blown fits, after which the patient lapsed into a coma and died. Seemingly unperturbed, he thought it desirable that these events should be 'presented as I observed them' - thus precipitating an outcry that cost him his job.

John Hughlings Jackson (1835-1911)

The great catalyst for this work, however, was the clinical studies of Hughlings Jackson. Jackson, the son of a wealthy Yorkshire farmer, was born at Green Hammerton just off the A1 outside York. He began his medical training at the now defunct medical school at York,[1] qualifying in 1856 and registering under the new act on the first day possible, January 1st. 1859. During his time at York, Jackson encountered two people who were to have a great influence on his future career. The first, **Thomas Laycock** (1812-1876), one of his tutors at York, had a considerable interest in neurology and was the first person to use bromides in the treatment of epilepsy. The second, **Jonathan Hutchinson** (1828-1913) of Selby is remembered for his eponymous description of the dilated pupil sometimes seen with raised intracranial pressure and of the triad of interstitial keratitis, notched teeth and labyrinthitis found in the then-common condition of congenital syphilis. Hutchinson, who was about seven years senior to Jackson at York, had moved to the London Hospital and it was he who persuaded his younger colleague to follow him to London.

The story of Jackson's appointment gives some indication of his strange, restless nature. Despite the fact that he was the only candidate he forgot to attend for interview and Hutchinson had to go off in a cab to round him up. But no sooner had he been appointed than he announced that he had decided to study philosophy instead. Exactly the same thing happened at the newly established Hospital for the Paralysed and Epileptic (Queen Square) where, to Hutchinson's disgust, he had fallen under the influence of Brown Sequard. Soon after obtaining an appointment there in 1862 he decided he did not like doing domiciliary visits and tendered his resignation. Fortunately he was talked out of both moves, but this sort of impulsive behaviour continued to be a hallmark of his character. It is said, for example, that he had never seen a play in one sitting, always walking out after one act and popping back a day or two later to see another. He was a voracious reader who would abandon dinner guests and retire to the fireside to read a book, yet his treatment of books was atrocious. Novels were torn in half for ease of transport and abandoned page by page as they were read, while his magnificent library was destroyed by his habit of tearing out pages of interest and sending them to colleagues.

Where medicine was concerned, Jackson was primarily a philosopher and a clinician. He had no interest in laboratory experiments, although he contended that the phenomena which he observed in minute detail - particularly focal fits due to cerebral tumours - 'should be considered as an anatomical and physiological experiment, although a rough one, on part of the brain'. Nor was his interpretation of these events simplistic, for while many believed that the phenomena produced or lost by seizures or ablation indicated the function of the damaged area, Jackson envisaged 'layers' of neural activity, loss of a higher level revealing the function of the level below. It was a complex idea, not made any easier by Jackson's literary style which, as one exasperated reviewer observed, was 'like the love of God, for it passeth all understanding'.

Be that as it may Jackson was, in the words of Sir Francis Walshe, 'a man who, using neither apparatus nor animal experiment, could nevertheless in the nineteenth century make fundamentally important contributions to neurophysiology by the application of scientific imagination to the material of his observations'. His genius was recognised by Charcot who coined the term Jacksonian epilepsy, pointing out that while the *phenomenon of* focal epilepsy had already been observed by his compatriot Bravais, the *significance* of such seizures had only now been appreciated. It was these observations which, in large measure, prompted the work for which the West Riding Lunatic Asylum was to become famous.

David Ferrier (1843-1928)

The scene was therefore set for the definitive scientific work, which was carried out by David Ferrier. Although Ferrier held clinical appointments he, unlike Jackson, was primarily a scientist. Graduating at Edinburgh in 1868 he soon obtained an M.D. (with gold medal) for a thesis on the corpora quadrigemina of various animals - studies conducted in a garden belonging to a G.P. in Bury St. Edmunds for whom he was working. He then moved to London where his attempts to continue his investigations in a shed in another garden in Upper Berkley Street were frustrated by anti-vivisectionists who, prior to the Cruelty to Animals Act of 1876, were becoming increasingly vociferous. It was therefore with some satisfaction that, in 1873, he was invited by his friend and fellow graduate Crichton Browne to continue his work at the West Riding Lunatic Asylum. Here he was given a laboratory (which is still standing - Fig. 6) and a 'liberal supply of guinea pigs, rabbits, cats and dogs'. Thus equipped he set about following up the work of Fritsch and Hitzig - which he felt was inconclusive - and 'putting to experimental proof the views entertained by Dr. Hughlings Jackson on the pathology of epilepsy, chorea and hemiparesis by imitating artificially the destroying and discharging lesions of the brain which his writings have defined and differentiated'.

In doing this work Ferrier had two great advantages. In the first place he was able to avoid the frogs and pigeons 'which have too often been the bane of clinical medicine', using - perhaps for

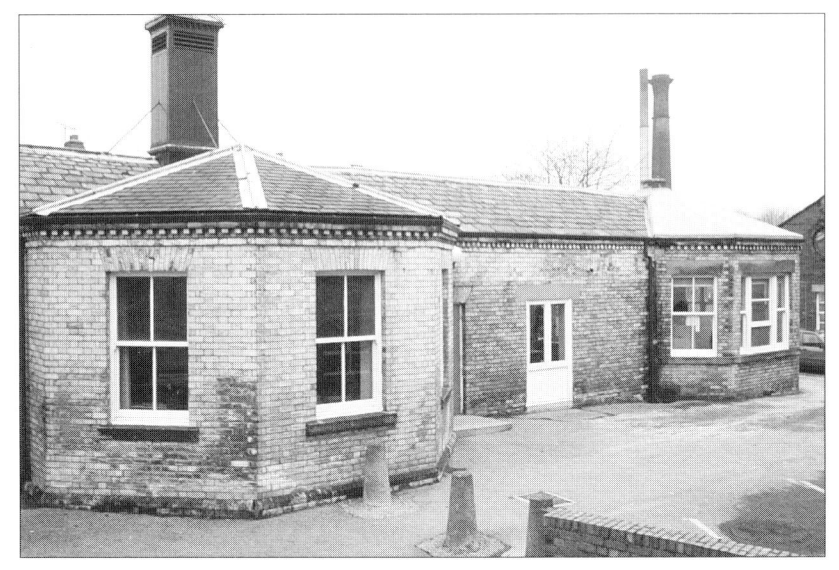

Fig. 6. The laboratory at Stanley Royd Hospital, Wakefield where Ferrier's work on cerebral localisation was done

the first time since Galen - apes bought with a grant from the Royal Society. Moreover, instead of the twitches with which earlier workers had to be satisfied he was able to use Faradic stimulation (introduced in 1870) to produce more sustained movements. Once started, the work proceeded with amazing speed. The idea was conceived in March 1873 and the first paper appeared (with one of Jackson's papers) in the Reports of the West Riding Lunatic Asylum later that year. By 1876 the work was finished and Ferrier had established beyond reasonable doubt that the phenomena produced by lesions of the cortex depend on their site and on whether they were irritative or destructive.

The presentation of the results

Although initially there was some dispute with the Royal Society, which felt that Fritch and Hitzig had not been given due credit for their work, Ferrier was invited to give the Croonian Lectures in 1874 and 1875 and was awarded the Fellowship in 1876. He also produced two books, dedicated respectively to

Jackson and to Charcot. But the most memorable event was the presentation of his findings at the seventh International Medical Conference in London in 1881. This spectacular meeting, to which 120,000 people, including all the crowned heads of Europe, were invited was opened by the Prince of Wales. It included 'an unusually abundant series of banquets, receptions and excursions', finishing with a feast at the Crystal Palace and a firework display with 'fire portraits' of Charcot and Sir James Paget. It was during the course of this conference that a famous meeting took place at which Goltz, Professor of Physiology at Strasbourg, and Ferrier presented their differing views. Goltz, who claimed that a dog from which the cerebral cortex had been removed was not physically impaired, produced such an animal for inspection. This creature, which so impressed the young Sherrington[2] that he decided to devote his life to neurophysiology, was killed and examined by a panel of experts and, later, by both Sherrington (who wrote his first paper on the subject) and Gordon Holmes. In the event the removal of the cortex proved to be less extensive than Goltz claimed. In his reply Ferrier argued that the effects of cortical ablation in lower animals may indeed be transient, and produced two monkeys. The first had been rendered deaf by the removal of parts of the temporal lobes. But it was the second monkey, from which one motor cortex had been removed, that created a sensation, for as this pathetic hemiplegic animal limped onto the rostrum, Charcot, one of the leading delegates, shouted 'C'est un malade!' The argument for cerebral localisation had been won.

Consequences

This demonstration had two major consequences. The first - the result of yet another attack by the antivivisectionists - was Ferrier's appearance in Bow Street Magistrates' Court on a charge of conducting 'fearful and shocking experiments without the authority of the Home Secretary.' From the outset Ferrier had in fact noted that 'before and during all these experiments ether or chloroform was administered', but it was true that following his clash with the anti-vivisectionists at Upper Berkley Street he had been refused a licence. However at the hearing, which was attended by a galaxy of scientific talent, it was successfully argued that the operations themselves were not done by Ferrier but by Professor Yeo, who had an appropriate qualification. The Times denounced the scandal which 'forced a British surgeon to go to a foreign country to do experiments that would benefit his patients' and both Charcot and Virchow poked fun at a nation which 'practices methods of hunting which far surpass in cruelty anything that is done in laboratories.' Overall an attempt to get a bit of cheap publicity seems to have rebounded on the heads of the anti-vivisectionists.

Ferrier's studies were, however, to have another consequence of more lasting significance. With the advent of anaesthesia in 1846 and of antiseptic surgery in 1867 a veritable explosion of surgical activity had taken place. This, however, did not incorporate 'the dark continent of the brain'. Indeed, as late as 1874 one leading surgeon affirmed that the skull 'will be forever closed to operations by the wise and humane surgeon'. Hitherto, of course, this was only reasonable, for the surgeon had had no means of ascertaining the site of the lesion on which he wished to operate. But knowing the function of various parts of the cortex he could now predict, from the nature of the patient's symptoms, where it lay and Ferrier wanted to know 'why surgeons, who fearlessly expose the abdominal viscera, shrink from opening the cranial cavity'. Not everyone was convinced that this was a good idea - indeed the Lancet commented that 'if Dr. Ferrier's suggestion meets with much practical response it is to be feared that cerebral localisation will soon have more to answer for than lives to boast of.' Others, however, were more adventurous. In 1876 Broca had located and drained a cerebral abscess that was causing aphasia and between 1876 and 1883 Macewen of Glasgow - to whom, according to Ferrier, 'the honour of having led the way in human neurosurgery' belonged - contrived to locate seven intracranial lesions of various sorts. Ferrier himself was finally able to see such an operation in 1884 when, at the Hospital for the Paralysed and Epileptic in Regent's Park (destroyed during the blitz) Rickman Godlee (Lister's nephew) removed a glioma which had been causing focal fits. The operation was watched by Jackson and Ferrier, and Crichton Browne dashed off a rather sickly letter to the Times extolling the fruits of physiological research. The public, preoccupied with the current attempt to rescue General Gordon from Khartoum, may not have noticed that the patient died of meningitis a few days later.

Two years after this Charcot himself, on another visit to England, saw a meningioma removed by Horsley. 'I held it in my hand', he told his students 'We must wonder at the doctrine of brain localisation which can give such results. One day everyone will start doing it.' His prediction was of course correct and in 1927, when Harvey Cushing was in London to give a review of his vast experience of neurosurgery he was introduced to a little old man whose name he failed, at first, to catch. To his delight he discovered that it was Ferrier, now 84 years old - the man whose studies in a Yorkshire asylum had laid the foundations on which the science of neurosurgery was built.

REFERENCES
Parsons, M. 'A scientific phrenology.' Leeds Medical School Postgraduate Diary, August 1991, 13.
Trotter, W. A landmark in modern neurology in Collected Papers, Oxford, 1941.

NOTES
1. The Medical School at York was founded in 1834, a year after the foundation of the York Medical Society. It had no buildings of its own, using instead the County Hospital (now a block of flats), the Dispensary, the Retreat and the York Philosophical Society (now the museum). Students, who paid the staff directly, could opt for 'sessional' or 'permanent' membership. As in many provincial centres the numbers were limited - never more than 20 per year. There was a suspicion that the institution was run more for the benefit of the staff than the students and as medicine became more technical it became impossible to maintain the service. It is said to have closed in 1859 but some teaching was still going on as late as 1867.
2. Twenty-five years later Sherrington was to dedicate his book *The Integrative Action of the Nervous System* to Ferrier 'In recognition of his many services to the physiology of the Central Nervous System.'

CHAPTER VIII

Industrial Medicine

Urbanisation and the growth of industry produced a host of new medical disorders, described in a classic work by the Leeds' surgeon Charles Turner Thackrah.

IT HAS BEEN known from very early times that certain occupations are associated with certain diseases. The Ancient World took little interest in such matters, however, for it did not regard workers as citizens and even Hippocrates, normally so concerned about the environment, tended to ignore these ailments. Industrial medicine, the study of occupational diseases, is therefore a relatively recent innovation.

The situation began to change in the sixteenth century when the metal mines of central Europe, which provided the coinage for the Continent, started to attract a number of visitors. Among these were two men, Georg Bauer and Paracelsus (himself a metallurgist), who described not only the process of mining but also ailments like mercury poisoning from which miners suffered. (Bauer also described the mischievous dwarfs that were supposed to infest the mines - a story which in due course was to become the basis of some of Grimm's fairy tales and, in more recent years, of Snow White and the seven (mining) dwarfs.) But industrial diseases were not studied in a systematic manner until 1700 when the University of Padua, which also produced the first great textbooks of anatomy (Vesalius) and of pathology (Morgagni), made its third great contribution to medicine. Written by Bernardino Ramazzini, *de Morbis Artificium Diatriba*, (which was translated into English by **Dr. Robert James** of Sheffield), surveyed the ill-effects of over 40 occupations and stressed the importance of preventative measures to safeguard the health of workers.

The problem of industrial diseases came to a peak in England during the Industrial Revolution when, from the middle of the eighteenth century, a large part of the rapidly expanding population moved from the country into the new manufacturing and mining centres of the North. Here, malnourished, overcrowded and working for long hours with toxic substances and dangerous machinery, they were a ready prey for infections, poisoning and injury. The plight of orphan child labourers, sent by the wagon-load from homes that were glad to be rid of the financial burden, was particularly sad. Leeds, which even before these developments was an important centre for textiles, saw its full measure of these problems. Between 1801 and 1831, largely as a result of the invention of the flying shuttle and the introduction of American cotton, its population had risen from 60,000 to 130,000 and by the start of the nineteenth century it was estimated that overall it housed 128 different trades. It was therefore hardly surprising that it should also produce the great British authority on industrial diseases, **Charles Turner Thackrah** (1795-1833).

Thackrah, the son of a local chemist, started work with a Leeds apothecary in 1811. To comply with new regulations he then went to Guy's Hospital in London where (as a fellow pupil of John Keats) he was taught by the renowned Astley Cooper. This was a crucial point in the history of British medicine, for under the influence of the great Parisian hospitals the emphasis of training had at last shifted from debate to 'observation of the diseased living, examination of the dead and experiments on living animals'. Thackrah was clearly a bright student, for he was awarded the prize offered by Astley Cooper. He was also a man of culture who was invited to give the inaugural lecture at the Leeds Philosophical and Literary Society. But sadly, at a time when consultants were elected (often after a little inducement) by the whole body of hospital subscribers, he was not sufficiently influential to obtain an appointment on the staff of The General Infirmary. Instead, in 1817, he was forced to accept the post of Town Surgeon, a lowly occupation which often went to the candidate prepared to accept the lowest salary. This failure, which he resented bitterly, nearly led to his downfall, but in the long run the appointment was to be the basis of his success.

Casting around for some means of improving his status Thackrah hit on the idea of teaching anatomy - a topic which, in those days, included what is now called physiology. This he was well qualified to do, for in addition to an excellent scientific training he had inherited something of Astley Cooper's dramatic manner. Within a short time he had developed a flourishing school in South Parade - an establishment which, like others of its type, depended heavily on the activities of 'resurrectionists'.[1] Here, still resentful of the staff of the Infirmary, he regaled his pupils with stories of their surgical incompetence and nepotistic appointments. These diatribes did not, of course, go unnoticed, and during the course of the ensuing feud one of Thackrah's pupils took a horse-whip to an apothecary from the Infirmary. At this stage Thackrah wrote an intemperate letter to the Leeds Mercury in which, among other things, he listed his qualifications and likened his opponents to 'skunks'. The dignified response from Mr. Samuel Smith, one of the surgeons involved, was prominently published on the front page of a later edition. After suggesting that Thackrah had used the incident to 'advertise your superior talents and unexampled persecution' it went on to point out that a doctor who had treated a well-bred young lady for 'ascites' when he, above all, was in a position to know the true cause of her rapidly expanding abdomen could hardly expect to be treated as a colleague by the rest of the profession.

It seems hardly possible that, after an incident of this sort, the two parties involved could be reconciled. But with all his faults Thackrah was clearly a gifted teacher and anatomist and four years later, in 1831, he was invited to join members of the staff of the Infirmary - including Mr Smith - to found the Leeds School of Medicine. It could indeed be argued that, for this purpose, they joined him, for it is recognised that Thackrah was 'the founder of academic training in Leeds'.

While these events were taking place, Thackrah had found that his lowly appointment as Town Surgeon was bringing him into contact with a wealth of virtually undiscovered clinical material, for less than 10% of the labouring population, with its 128 different trades, could be described as truly healthy. From well-known establishments like the mills, the potteries and the foundry through to coffee-roasters, snuff makers and tailors (who were so prone to anal fistula that they founded their own fistula club) the work, the working conditions and the home circumstances of the labouring classes produced a seemingly endless variety of medical problems. Thackrah was able not only to record these conditions but also, using techniques recently introduced in the Parisian school, to study their symptoms and to analyse them statistically.

His results, the first survey of its sort in English, were published in 1831 in a book entitled *The Effects of the Principal Arts, Trades and Professions and of Civic States and Habits of Living on Health and Longevity; with a particular reference to The Trades and Manufactures of Leeds*. It was enthusiastically received and was reprinted in America almost at once. This book was rapidly followed by an equally successful publication on an outbreak of cholera in Newcastle - a condition of which Thackrah had a considerable knowledge following an outbreak in Leeds in 1825 - and then, in 1832, by a second, enlarged edition of his treatise on industrial diseases. In preparing this he had visited Manchester and Hull and had sought the opinion of his many students. His book was to play a major part in the reform of working conditions - a triumph which Thackrah was not to see for a year later he died of tuberculosis at the comparatively early age of 38.[2]

To illustrate the nature of industrial diseases it is worth looking in a little more detail at three which have a particular connection with this area. The first, anthrax, is a bacillary infection which can invade the skin to cause a 'malignant pustule' or the lungs to cause woolsorters' disease, a serious systemic disorder which, even with antibiotics, can still be fatal.. Thackrah, who said that 'the occupation of woolsorter produces no sensible effect on health', was unaware of these conditions for they were only introduced into England in the second half of the nineteenth century on wool and mohair from the middle East and India. As was so often the case, it was the workers themselves who first recognised what came to be known as the *maladie de Bradford*. They were indeed so sure of the cause that it became customary to draw lots as to who should handle certain fleeces. Direct contact was not, however, necessary, and at least one secretary who merely walked through the sorting sheds, which were so dusty that it was often impossible to see from one end to the other, died of the disease.

The impact of these events within a relatively small community was immense and in February 1878 a letter appeared in the Bradford Observer which read: 'Sir, Within a month three woolsorters have died from blood poisoning contracted in the same shed of the same factory in Manchester Road. Occasional deaths from blood poisoning .... may perhaps be inevitable; but the recurrence within so short a time of three such cases suggests either that the wool itself or the shed is specially un-wholesome. May I hope for your help to induce manufacturers to remedy all that is remediable in this deadly trade ......'. The plea soon began to bear fruit. It had been suggested by **Dr. J E Eddison** of Leeds that the condition might be related to anthrax, a lethal disease of animals found in many parts of the world, and this idea was confirmed by **Dr. J H Bell**, a Bradford G.P., who contrived to transmit the disease from man to animals. Attempts to contain the problem were, however, unsuccessful and in 1905 another Bradford G.P., **Dr. F W Eurich** (1867-1945) (who probably wrote the letter quoted above) was asked by a joint board of the Bradford Chamber of Commerce and the Operatives Association to look into the matter.[3]

At this time bacteriology was still in its infancy and Eurich was well aware that the meticulous work he was about to undertake, which went on for 15 years, was exceedingly dangerous. It was also poorly paid and very time-consuming, for apart from being done on top of his duties as a general practitioner the Bradford Health Department refused to allow him to do animal experiments, despite intense local interest in the condition. These therefore had to be carried out in the Medical School at Leeds, where Eurich was later to become Professor of Forensic Pathology. But it was as a result of his painstaking studies that the nature of the condition was confirmed, an efficient (Eurich's) method of disinfecting imported fleeces was introduced and the disease was eradicated.

The second topic of local interest is the dust disease, asbestosis. This condition, which causes fibrosis of the lungs that can undergo malignant change, is mentioned because the UK manufacturers of asbestos had a branch factory, J W Roberts, in Armley, Leeds. This establishment, which is said to have caused widespread pollution of the district, is the subject of intensive and ongoing litigation. By as early as the 1920's the problem had become known to **Matthew Stewart** (1885-1945), Professor of Pathology at Leeds, who had been asked to do autopsies on a number of the firm's employees. Stewart was one of the first to realise that the condition could be associated with cancer, but his attempts to set up a Medical Research Council trial were inhibited - partly, it is supposed, for fear that the results might cause still more unemployment in the inter-war years. His extensive research was however given little publicity, a fact which has caused some disquiet as his services were retained at an early stage by the company involved.

The third group of workers is not exclusively linked with Yorkshire, but has got an interesting historical association. 'Climbing boys' sent to explore and clear the labyrinthine chimneys of Victorian houses were of course liable to falls and to asphyxiation in soot.[4] But in 1775 Percival Pott pointed out that sweeps were also prone to develop cancer of the scrotum. Over a century later it was realised that contact with mineral oils, as for example in mule spinners, had the same effect and that carcinomas could be induced experimentally by painting the skin with coal tar or shale oil. This subject was studied by **Dr. Sydney Henry**, a cancer specialist at the Royal Free Hospital and one of H.M. Inspectors of Factories who served on the 1928 inquiry into asbestos-related problems at Armley. Subsequently Dr. Henry developed an almost obsessional interest in chimney sweeps and their activities and built up a large collection of photographs relating to all aspects of the trade. This collection is now housed in the Leeds' City Art Gallery.

REFERENCES
Hunter, D. Health in Industry. Penguin 1959.
Meikeljohn, A. Charles Turner Thackrah. Livingstone 1957.

NOTES
1. Bodysnatching was common in and around Leeds. Indeed one Wakefield family is said to have made its fortune when, in the course of digging an exceptionally deep grave to protect the remains of a relative, they struck a rich seam of coal.
2. His grave, hitherto unknown, was recently re-discovered by Dr. Graham Hardy in St. John's Churchyard, Dewsbury Moor (Fig. 7).
3. Eurich's father, the German representative of a Bradford textile firm, was among the many Germans who sought refuge in Bradford prior to the First World war. Despite his untiring efforts on behalf of the community Eurich himself was to be persecuted for this connection during that conflict.

4. In view of St. Nicholas' propensities for climbing chimneys and for saving small boys it was appropriate that an annual dinner should have been held for 100 apprentice sweeps in the sweeps' church, St. George the Martyr, Queen Square, London, on the feast of St. Nicholas, December 25th.

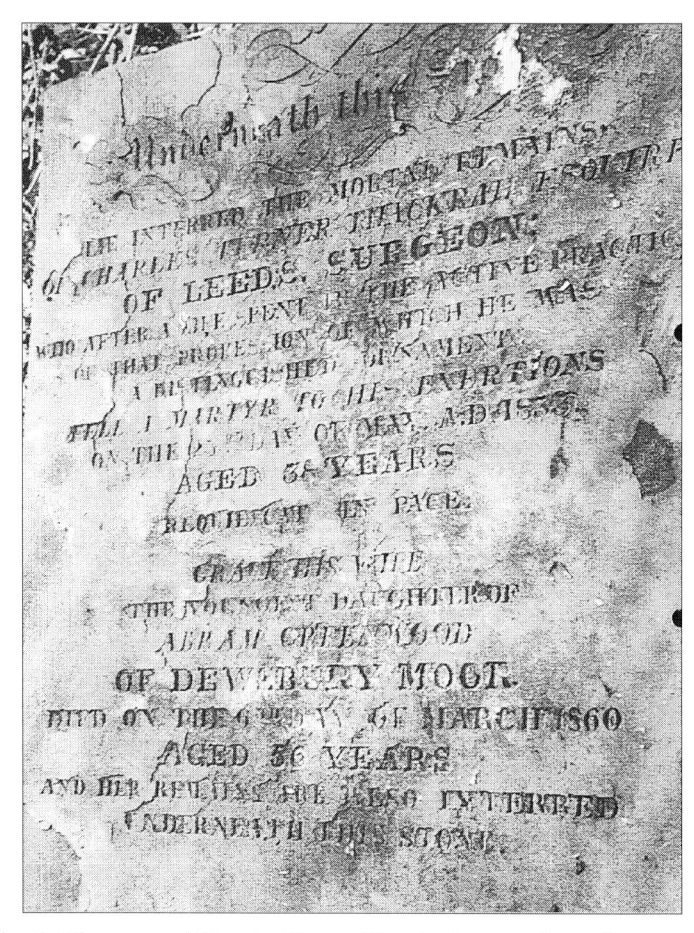

Fig. 7. The grave of Charles Turner Thackrah, recently re-discovered in St. John's Churchyard, Dewsbury Moor.
(By kind permission of Dr. Graham Hardy)

CHAPTER IX

The Leeds Anatomy Riots – 1832

Eighteen thirty-two was an eventful year in the history of Leeds. The eagerly awaited Reform Bill had at last become law, but the wild rejoicing of the proletariat ended abruptly when it discovered that it had been outwitted, not once, but twice. To begin with the aristocracy had neatly averted rebellion by enfranchising and allying themselves with the middle classes, thus driving a wedge between these two groups and the poor, who gained nothing. Worse still, during the turmoil associated with the passage of the Reform Bill their erstwhile allies had spirited the Anatomy Act through Parliament, a measure designed to prevent 'bodysnatching' by the simple expedient of using the bodies of paupers instead. It was not therefore to be expected that the doctors and reformers who invaded the slums during the 1832 epidemic of cholera - or the supporter of the Anatomy Act who appeared as a Parliamentary candidate - would be greeted with affection.

The Reform Bill

IN THE EARLY years of the nineteenth century England, like the rest of Europe, was in a state of political turmoil. It was indeed feared that a combination of rural poverty and agitation in the new cities created by the Industrial Revolution might precipitate a rebellion like the one which had just occurred in France. The Tories, whose instinctive response to such troubles was one of repression, had fallen from power and even the Whigs had been forced to deport four hundred farm-workers to restore order in the south-east of the country. They were however able to recognise that there were at least two components in the current agitation. On the one hand there was the 'revolutionary' proletariat, with whom they had little sympathy. But there was also a middle class element which, having created the lucrative new industries, deeply resented the fact that it had no political representation. Calculating that if the demands of the latter group were to be met the situation might be defused, they introduced the first Reform Bill.

Reform was long overdue, for although the Lords seemed to take little part in government they had in fact retained a large measure of control over the Commons. The Duke of Buckingham alone, for example, could command twelve votes from relatives and pocket boroughs, while great industrial cities like Manchester and Leeds had no representatives at all. The first objective of the Bill was therefore to obtain a more equitable distribution of seats by re-allocating 150 of those currently assigned to rotten boroughs. The second was to extend the franchise to the middle class - a group demarcated by their ability to pass the 'ten pound householder' qualification devised by Baines[1] in a survey conducted in Leeds in 1831. In practice the effect of these changes was to be more apparent than real, for the poor were entirely excluded and the influence of the 'upper class' was far from extinct. Nevertheless the measure was widely acclaimed by the public. It was however defeated and in the ensuing election - in which Reform was the only issue - the Whigs were returned with an immense majority. But although two further bills passed through the Commons with ease, both were rejected by the Lords. A constitutional crisis seemed inevitable until, faced with scenes of wild public disorder and a threat that the Lords would be 'packed' with supporters, opponents of the Reform Bill decided to abstain. In 1832 it became law.

The Anatomy Act

During this upheaval a second, entirely unrelated bill was also working its way onto the statute book. Since the beginning of the eighteenth century there had been a steady increase in the number of cadavers dissected in hospitals and schools of anatomy. Such bodies could of course be obtained from the gallows, for under the Murder Act of 1752 a judge could decree that a particularly vile offender should not only be hanged, but also that his body should be dissected in public and denied a burial service or burial. There was, however, a gross discrepancy between the number of bodies made available in this way - about twelve a year in London - and the hundreds that were being dissected. The rest were simply stolen.

The theft of bodies for dissection was as old as anatomy itself, and for many years doctors had participated in these episodes. But although, by comparison with those stealing game, offenders were dealt with leniently, a series of judgements given towards the end of the eighteenth century had shown that doctors could no longer expect to be exonerated by the courts. From the turn of the century, therefore, schools of anatomy were supplied almost entirely by gangs of professional 'body-snatchers'. In Leeds, for example, there was **Thomas Hodgson**, who lived near the Golden Cross Inn at Sheepscar in a group of cottages known (until they were demolished) as Resurrection Row. Between 1820 and 1832 he is thought to have supplied anatomists such as Hey and Thackrah with as many as twelve bodies annually and they spoke on his behalf when he appeared in court. They may indeed have funded his medical studies in Edinburgh University (which he never completed) after he 'retired'. But Hodgson and his associates also ran a thriving 'export' business, and at various times bodies were found on coaches destined for Manchester, Newcastle and Edinburgh and on ships sailing from Selby and Hull. Amazingly, although he appeared in court on at least three occasions, the longest sentence he received was twelve months' imprisonment - at a time when those caught stealing game might be deported.

The authorities, who were well aware of such activities, were reluctant to intervene. They recognised the need for training in anatomy, but shied away from the unpopular task of designating the large number of bodies needed for this purpose. Instead, they tried to ensure that supplies were maintained by ignoring the looting of hospital mortuaries, providing additional cadavers from the great military hospitals and discouraging the interception of bodies imported from elsewhere. The public, by contrast, did everything in its power to bring the practice to an end. The depth of graves was increased and they were surrounded with traps and markers. Stouter coffins - some made of metal - were introduced and funerals were deferred until putrefaction would have rendered the corpse useless. Graves were covered with stone slabs or metal 'mortsafes' and graveyards were guarded, often from specially constructed watch-towers. One man even ordered his heirs - on pain of being disinherited - to place his coffin in the rafters of his barn in

Stevenage, where it remains to this day. To a large extent these measures were successful, and as a result cadavers became more scarce and considerably more expensive. Students began to find that it was cheaper to train on the Continent (where there was an abundance of material) and English schools of anatomy were threatened with insolvency. Then, to complete the disaster, two judicial rulings made it clear that even causing a body to be stolen, or receiving a body knowing it to have been stolen was a punishable offence. If the teaching of anatomy was to continue, new legislation would have to be introduced.

It was probably the surgeon Abernethy who, in 1819, first suggested that the bodies of paupers should be used. After all, as cynics observed, it was from the shallow multiple graves of paupers, with their flimsy coffins, that the bulk of the bodies was already obtained. There was also a growing feeling - presently to be reflected in the Poor Law Bill of 1834 - that the 'undeserving poor' were guilty of some sort of crime. There was therefore much support for Bentham's idea that those maintained by the state should repay their debt to the state - with their bodies. This, it was suggested, need not cause distress if only 'unclaimed' bodies were to be used.- an observation which ignored the fact that those who claimed the body (who had to be near relatives) were then faced with the cost of a funeral they could not afford. The distress caused to those whose mortal remains were under discussion, who could anticipate an ignominious end hitherto reserved for the worst sort of murderers, was simply ignored. So also was the suggestion that other people maintained by the state - the monarchy, members of parliament and the holders of innumerable sinecures - might also 'repay their debt to society' in this way, along with the surgeons and anatomists who supported this worthy cause.

The first Bill 'for Preventing the Unlawful Disinterment of Human Bodies and for Regulating Schools of Anatomy', which enshrined these ideas, was drawn up by a carefully selected committee and eased through the Commons with such skill that it was dubbed the Midnight Bill by its opponents. It was however defeated in the Lords where, in July 1829, a group of peers which included the **Earl of Harewood** successfully insisted that the poor had a right to a decent burial. But between the report of the Select Committee in July 1828 and the rejection of the Bill a year later there had been another sinister development - murder. This was not entirely unforeseen, for Bentham had warned Peel that if a sufficient number of cadavers was not forthcoming, the deficit might be made good in this way. The discovery that Burke and Hare (who were not in fact body-snatchers) had killed and sold sixteen people in Edinburgh simply confirmed his misgivings. In 1831 a second pair of 'burkers' - Bishop and Williams - was arrested in London and it was estimated by Wakley, the reforming editor of The Lancet, that the number of people who had died in this way probably ran into three figures. Faced with these revelations the general public, already incensed by the violation of graveyards and the rejection of the Reform Bill, turned in fury on doctors and anatomists.

Prompted by this outcry, and under cover of the on-going battle about Reform, Warburton introduced a second bill. Although couched in simpler, less emotive language - for the title made no mention of graveyards and dissection was referred to as 'examination' - its purpose was nevertheless unchanged. Indeed, as the peer who introduced it to the Upper House naively complained, 'it would be an improvement if the provisions could be so framed as not to point out so disturbingly that its operation had reference to a particular class'. In one respect it was an improvement, for it did abolish the dissection of those executed for murder - a practice which discredited doctors and fostered the popular horror of anatomy. But it also had major defects. It was assumed, for example, that a body could be used for dissection unless the patient had registered his objection (a policy again suggested in recent times in connection with the 'donation' of organs for transplantation). But as opponents pointed out, even such paupers as were aware of the provision rarely had any means of recording their wishes. Conversely, the master of the workhouse was under no obligation to provide bodies, a fact which was to cause considerable difficulties in certain areas. The Bill also failed to prohibit the sale of bodies, perhaps because this was an important source of income to anatomists (who sold 'parts' of bodies to students) or even because Warburton was himself a shareholder in the new London University School of Anatomy. And the obligation to provide a Christian burial left anatomists in some doubt, as recent events have shown, as to whether they could retain specimens. Nevertheless, in August 1832 the Bill became law.

In Leeds, as elsewhere, the provisions of the new Act were carefully examined. Already disappointed by their failure to benefit from the Reform Bill the poor were incensed to find that the very people they had supported so vociferously had now produced another measure which treated their cherished customs and their very remains with utter contempt. These feelings surfaced in October 1832, two months after the Act came into force, when the Trustees of the Workhouse expressed their approval of it, criticised the theft of bodies from graveyards and appointed a committee to supervise the distribution of cadavers. However, there was only a majority of one vote in favour of these motions and two days later a further proposal was passed directing that notices should be posted in every ward of the workhouse advising the 'friendless poor' of their predicament and telling them 'how to prevent their bodies being given to the schools of anatomy for dissection'. A month later, at a tumultuous meeting to appoint Trustees for the coming year, opponents of the Act had a further victory. All those who had voted in favour of dissection were disqualified and a new board entirely opposed to it was elected. Supporters who tried to expound the virtues of anatomy and the (very questionable) benefits its study would bestow on the poor were howled down amidst demands for a measure that would 'dispense equal justice to all - fat sinecurists as well as the worn-out labourer'. The dispute spilt over into the December election and the newly appointed Inspector of Anatomy wrote in alarm to an anatomist in Leeds and to Baines, the editor of the Leeds Mercury, seeking information. His intervention must have had some effect, for a few weeks later he reported that the School of Anatomy had obtained at least one body and had 'every prospect of obtaining greater supplies'. Unrest continued, however, with an attack on an anatomy school in Hull in 1834 and the destruction of the school in Sheffield in 1835.

Cholera

The timing of the second Anatomy Bill was doubly unfortunate for, in addition to the unrest caused by the failure of the Reform Bill, the country was in the throes of an epidemic of cholera. The disease had spread from the Far East and through Russia, arriving in Hull in 1831. It extended rapidly, and the following year 1817 cases were reported in Leeds with 702 deaths. Historically this outbreak was of some importance, for at the time the cause of the infection was unknown.[2] But detailed plans drawn up by the Poor Law medical officer for Leeds, **Robert Baker**, showed clearly that cases tended to cluster round the streams draining into the River Aire. Further observations - which were to be incorporated by Edwin Chadwick in his *Report of the Sanitary Condition of the Labouring Population of Great Britain* - revealed that the residents in these areas were living in conditions of the utmost squalor. Boot and Shoe Yard, for example, a cul-de-sac near Kirkgate, was found to have 340 residents in its 34 houses and 'at least twice that number during periods of haytime and harvest' - an indication of how close the countryside was to the centre of the town in the nineteenth century. The area, which had not been cleaned for years, was covered with 'a surface of human excrement' and seventy-five cartloads of manure were removed. Worse still the basements in this district, which was virtually devoid of drains, were regularly inundated when the River Aire was in flood, distributing this filth in all directions. Yet these properties were said to pay 'the best income of any in the borough'.

In the circumstances of the time this new epidemic fuelled the well-established atmosphere of resentment and mistrust. Victims were being forcibly removed to hospitals - which many believed were used by doctors to experiment on their poorer patients. Those who died were hastily buried, so that well established rituals could not be observed. Bodies were often buried in remote and even unconsecrated graveyards, from which they could easily be stolen and the homes of the poor were invaded by inspectors of various sorts, poking about for no evident reason. For a restless population, resentful of authority in general and of doctors in particular, it was a further source of irritation which precipitated riots in Leeds and several other centres.

The Leeds' Anatomy Riots

Matters came to a head in December 1832 when, for the first time, the citizens of Leeds met to nominate candidates for parliament. The Tory candidate was Michael Sadler, a respected local linen merchant whose sponsorship of factory reform had endeared him to the proletariat. Indeed some, perhaps bewildered by the new procedure, saw no need for 'Toaries and Redigals and such like while Oastler and Sadler and them'll stand up for us'. Stand up, that is, against the likes of the Liberal candidate John Marshall who, as heir to the largest flax mill in Europe, was one of the main local employers. But it was the second Liberal candidate whose presence roused the anger of the mob. Unlike his colleagues Thomas Babington Macaulay,[3] a professional politician, was a stranger to Leeds. Previously member for the pocket borough of Calne, he had lost his seat as a result of the Reform Bill and had been imported by Baines as someone who would represent the town with distinction. So far his experiences of Leeds had been agreeable, for the 'very honest, substantial manufacturers' entertaining him - no doubt well aware of the value of influence - were anxious to meet his every wish. Macaulay, however, had yet to meet the mob, and if he did not know Leeds, Leeds - with the battle to block the provisions of the Anatomy Act fresh in its mind - certainly knew him. For Macaulay had been one of the sponsors of the Act.

Nineteenth century elections were always boisterous, but it was a particularly turbulent procession that set off to escort the Tory candidate. It had two banners. The first, which showed poorly clad children struggling to work through the snow, was clearly aimed at Marshall. But it was the second Tory banner, which had a yellow (Liberal) border, that was to become the hallmark of the occasion. It depicted a skeleton bearing a scroll on which were written the words 'Anatomy Bill to better the condition of the helpless poor', and the subscription 'Macaulay and the Anatomy Bill' (Fig. 8). In the imagery of the time this was taken to mean that Macaulay, stripped of his clothes, was exactly the same as the paupers he wished to exploit or even - as in the medieval dance of death - that he was Death itself, leading victims to their inevitable fate. Either way it was clearly deeply offensive, and strenuous but unsuccessful attempts were made to capture it. But although Sadler's supporters included several doctors the majority, as Oastler pointed out, 'did not live in ten pound houses' and therefore had no votes. The fact that Marshall and Macaulay were returned has, however, been forgotten. The lasting memorial of this year of turmoil, and of Leeds' first parliamentary election, was the banner with the skeleton.

REFERENCES

Anning, S.T. Leeds House of Recovery. Medical History 1969. 13. 226.
Bryant, A. English Saga. Collins 1940. 19.
Churchill, W.S. The Great Democracies. Cassell 1956. 36-41.

Fernando, N. and Puntis, J. The Leeds cholera epidemic of 1832. Yorkshire Medicine 2001. No. 2. 42.

Fraser, D. A History of Modern Leeds,Manchester 1980. 276.

Green, M.A. Bodysnatching in West Yorkshire. Yorkshire Medicine Autumn 1989. 20.

Kerr, K. The York cholera epidemic of 1832. Yorkshire Medicine 1994. No3. 18.

Richardson, R. Death, Dissection and the Destitute. Penguin 1988.

NOTES

1. Editor of the Leeds Mercury and father-in-law of the neurologist W E Gowers.
2. It was not until 1854 that Snow stopped the epidemic in Soho by disabling the local pump.
3. Better known for his *History of England* and the *Lays of Ancient Rome*.

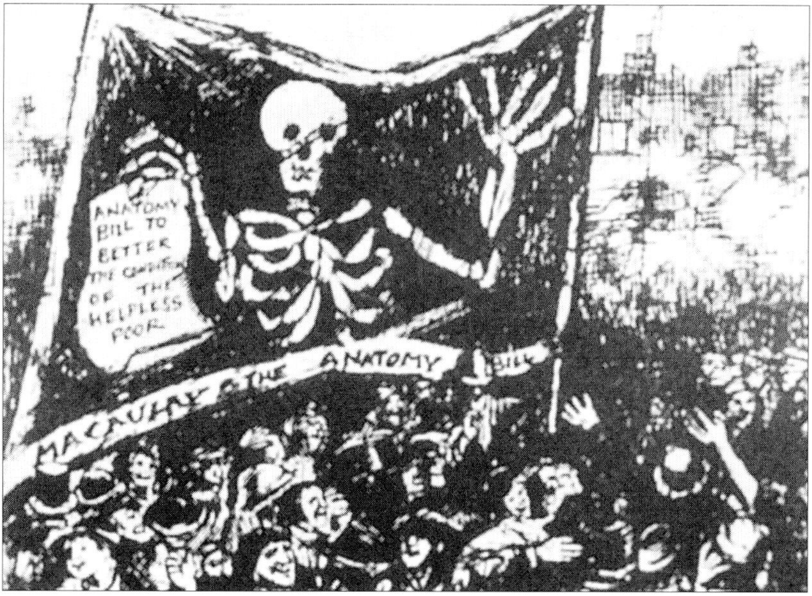

Fig. 8. Cartoon of the banner attacking Thomas Macaulay, a sponsor of the Anatomy Act, carried at the election in Leeds 1832.

CHAPTER X

The Development of Anaesthesia

Yorkshire has many links with the development of anaesthesia, including a dramatic early attempt to use an artificial ventilator.

ALTHOUGH THE eighteenth century saw major developments in the arts, sciences and technology it is noticeable that for the most part these were made, not by the Universities and the established Church, but by well informed individuals. **Joseph Priestley** (1733-1804) was a prime example of such men. Born in Fieldhead, Birstall, near Leeds he was denied access to the English Universities because he was a nonconformist. This however was to his advantage, for while the Universities were petrified the academy at Daventry, which accepted Dissenters, was able to provide him with a sound, forward-looking education that fired his interest in science. Consequently, although he entered the church (and became embroiled in various religious controversies), it is for his scientific achievements that he is chiefly known. While working in Nantwich he started a class that was so popular in the locality that he was invited to join the staff of the well-known Dissenting college at Warrington. Here his classes were regarded as a major innovation, and it was through the influence of one of his many pupils who went on to Edinburgh that he was awarded the degree of Doctor of Laws at that University. He also had contacts with the scientific fraternity in London, where he spent a month each year, and in 1766 he was made a Fellow of the Royal Society.

In 1767, the year in which the General Infirmary was founded, Priestley returned to Leeds as minister of the Mill Hill Chapel in City Square - the church where Lord Moran was married. Hitherto his studies had been mainly in the fields of electricity and optics but now, in a series of experiments 'in which only Mr. Hey,[1] a surgeon at the Infirmary, showed much interest', he turned his attention to the relatively unexplored topic of gases. He observed 'fixed air' (CO_2) produced during fermentation in the brewery next to his home - a substance which, 50 years later, Henry Hickman was to proffer (fortunately without success) as an anaesthetic because it caused 'suspended animation' in animals. In a famous experiment recalled by his statue in the City Square at Leeds he showed that by heating mercuric oxide he could produce 'dephlogisticated air' - a gas which supported life and combustion and which Lavoisier re-named oxygen. And among a number of other gases he isolated nitrous oxide.

Some thirty years later Humphry Davy, an apothecary's assistant, showed that inhalation of nitrous oxide caused giggling and dizziness and the substance acquired the name of 'laughing gas'. He demonstrated its effect to various friends including Coleridge and Southey, who wrote 'Davy has invented a new pleasure for which language has no name. I am going for more this evening .....'. Yet sadly, despite a crying need for something to relieve the agony of operations, no attention was paid to Davy's more important observations that nitrous oxide would relieve pain, that (mixed with oxygen) it caused reversible unconsciousness in animals and that 'it might probably be used with advantage during surgery'. As is so often the case the medical profession was lamentably slow in exploiting an important discovery and it was not until December 1844 that Horace Wells, having seen 'Professor' Gardner Colton demonstrate laughing gas at a fair, volunteered to have a molar tooth extracted while under its influence. This successful experiment was repeated several times but, to Wells' distress, failed when he tried to demonstrate it in John Warren's dentistry class. Wells' subsequent history was tragic, for he became depressed and addicted to chloroform, was arrested for throwing sulphuric acid at two prostitutes and killed himself while in prison.

Nitrous oxide was not, of course, the first anaesthetic substance to be used for surgery or indeed for entertainment. Once more, it may have been experience with 'ether frolics' that led William Clarke and Crawford Long independently to use this drug - which had been known for 300 years - for dental and minor surgical procedures. Curiously these successful experiments, done in 1842, were not reported at that time and the definitive tests did not take place until October 1846 when Charles Jackson - a man more interested in geology than in medicine - encouraged Thomas Morton (who had worked with Wells) to test a mixture of air and ether on a domestic pet, on himself and eventually on a patient. He then persuaded Warren to try this anaesthetic on two further patients. At that stage Morton unfortunately lost all credibility when, instead of publicising the successful results, he tried to disguise the colour and smell of the ether and claimed that he was using a new gas, letheon. When this subterfuge failed he and Jackson resorted to litigation over the question of who invented the idea of using ether. The upshot, once more, was tragic, for Morton died in poverty and Jackson in an asylum.

News of the use of ether was publicised by Henry Bigelow on November 18th 1846 and within a month it had been successfully employed in Paris and London. Leeds, always renowned for its surgery, cannot have been far behind, for 'during the winter session of 1846/7' a group of students began to experiment in the dissecting room of the medical school on East Parade, within sight of Priestley's church. One of them, **Claudius Galen Wheelhouse**, described how 'we rigged up a large glass vase, like a tea urn, filled with sponges, attached an india rubber tube to the spout, saturated the sponges with aether and through the tube inhaled the vapour as though it was a Turkish hookah pipe, and we fell over one after another quite insensible and unconscious of anything that was done to us ...... before many days we saw patients operated on in this insensible condition, and we found that they recovered quite as well as those who had borne the agony of their operation'. Curiously one of the most ardent advocates of anaesthesia at the Infirmary was **Thomas Nunneley** (1809-1870), a man who, a few years later, was to launch a violent and entirely irrational attack on the next great innovation, antiseptic surgery.

Ether, however, was not without its problems, for it had an offensive smell, was irritant and worked slowly and in 1847 Flourens suggested that chloroform, discovered some 15 years earlier, might be more satisfactory. This drug was pioneered by Simpson in Edinburgh who, along with friends who were testing new agents, is said to have been found unconscious beneath a table on which some had been spilt. It came to prominence, however, as a result of the work of another Yorkshireman, **John Snow** (1813-1858). Snow was born in North St., York and trained at Newcastle.

He then worked for eighteen months as an assistant to a Mr. Warburton at Pateley Bridge before returning to York where he seems to have spent much of his time founding a temperance society. (Snow was an ardent teetotaller and during the cholera epidemic in Soho he was dismayed to find that the local brewers, who had their own uncontaminated supplies of fluid, were immune to the outbreak he successfully curtailed). By the age of 23 he had moved on to London and it was here that he began to experiment, first with ether and then with chloroform. In 1850 he attended the birth of one of Queen Victoria's children and three years later, at the birth of Prince Leopold, he gave chloroform with great success. Strangely, having established a lasting reputation in two entirely different fields of medicine, his death at the age of 44 was barely noticed by the Lancet, although a large treatise on the use of chloroform helped, posthumously, to bring his name to prominence.

The debate about the relative risks of the various forms of anaesthesia continued and by degrees it became evident that chloroform, for all its virtues, was the most dangerous of the three. This was shown in 1896 when, in an early form of audit, it was decreed that all anaesthetic deaths at the General Infirmary at Leeds had to be reported to the Board. In every case in which the name of the agent responsible is given the drug involved was chloroform, which was implicated in at least six deaths among 3,800 operations over a 15 month period at this time. These deliberations resulted, in 1896, in the appointment of the first professional anaesthetists at the Infirmary, one of whom was to introduce the Rowling chloroform bottle, named after **Samuel Rowling** (1874-1950).

Yorkshire therefore had links with the development of all three of the main anaesthetics, for it saw the discovery of nitrous oxide and the early trials of ether and was associated with the promoter of chloroform. These, however, were not its only contributions to the development of anaesthesia, for Yorkshire also witnessed the first significant trial of a muscle relaxant (a drug used to facilitate surgery by relaxing the muscles of the chest or abdominal wall) and of its use with intermittent positive pressure (assisted) respiration.

Like Priestley, **Charles Waterton** (1782-1865) was a friend of William Hey. Hey had indeed bled him during a bout of pneumonia - a technique which Waterton learned and practised for the remainder of his life. Again like Priestley, he was excluded from the English Universities by his faith, in this instance Catholicism - not that this was a matter of great importance, for Waterton's preferred methods of learning were by personal observation and experience. He was an authority on natural history, both in this country and in South America where his family had estates, and his home at Walton Hall near Wakefield was a nature reserve and a museum for exotic animals which, with great skill, he had preserved. His contribution to anaesthesia, however, stemmed from an interest in the poison curare (or, as he called it, wourali) used on blowpipe darts by natives of Guyana. This substance had in fact been imported in 1584 by Sir Walter Raleigh but was overshadowed by his other discovery, the potato. It had also been studied by Benjamin Brodie, who received the Copley medal of the Royal Society in 1811. But Waterton's experience was even more profound, for he had witnessed the (very peaceful) death of a hunter accidentally wounded by one of these weapons Following this he contrived, with some difficulty, to watch its preparation and to obtain samples of the material which are now in the School of Medicine at Leeds. After unsuccessfully trying simple measures to preserve the lives of birds injected with wourali he resorted (in 1814) to a more elaborate technique of which he had heard. Having purchased a three-year-old donkey from a London sweep he injected it with the drug and ten minutes later the animal appeared to be dead. He then made an incision in the trachea and started to inflate the lungs with bellows - a technique already used by Vesalius, Hooke and Lettsom's Royal Humane Society but without, of course, the administration of curare. Two hours later the animal started to move but it was four hours before this primitive form of intermittent positive pressure ventilation could be discontinued. The donkey - named Wourali - made a complete recovery and lived for 25 years on the Walton Hall estate.

This experience suggested to Waterton that wourali might be of value in the treatment of hydrophobia (rabies), a condition which, at that time, was not uncommon in Great Britain. One of the most distressing of all diseases, it caused spasms of such intensity that euthanasia (for example by suffocation between two feather beds) was thought by some to be justifiable. Indeed a passage by Axel Munthe suggests that Pasteur himself 'helped to a painless death' a group of Russian peasants who were in an advanced stage of the disease. Even if it did not cure the condition, it seemed that wourali might at least relieve the victim of these dreadful spasms and it was therefore with some enthusiasm that Waterton responded to an invitation from the Nottingham medical community to see a policeman with hydrophobia in 1839. Sadly the patient died before he arrived, although during his visit his hosts prevailed on him to repeat his experiment on two more donkeys.

In 1844 Claude Bernard, who knew of Waterton's studies, showed that after injection of curare he was able to do what he called a 'physiological autopsy' on animals whose internal organs were still functioning normally. He also discovered that, whereas the muscles responded normally to stimulation, stimulation of the motor nerves had no effect. He therefore concluded that curare acted on (and only on) the motor nerves - an error pointed out by his pupil Vulpian who correctly suggested that its action was actually on the recently discovered motor end-plates. It was, however, to be almost a century before this observation was put to practical use in surgery and it was not until 1954 that **Hugh Garland, John Ablett** and others opened a tetanus unit at the General Infirmary at Leeds where patients with this condition, which in some ways resembles hydrophobia, were successfully treated with Waterton's regime of paralysis and intermittent positive pressure respiration.

REFERENCES

Ashcroft, A. John Snow, Victorian physician. in Medicine in Northumbria, Pybus Society,1993.
Nelson, G.A. Charles Waterton. University of Leeds Medical Journal 1957.6.54.
Puntis, J. Joseph Priestley and Medicine. Yorkshire Medicine Autumn 1996, 30.

NOTES
1. Priestley was later to propose Hey for the Fellowship of the Royal Society.

CHAPTER XI

The General Infirmary at Leeds

The introduction of civic hospitals in the eighteenth century was an important step in the growth of English medicine. The second Infirmary at Leeds was also a landmark in the design of hospitals.

THE CREATION of civic hospitals was one of the unsung benefits of the Industrial Revolution. At the beginning of the eighteenth century England had few such buildings, for the great monastic foundations which continued to serve this purpose on the continent had been dissolved by Henry VIII and the so-called 'hospitals' that remained were mostly small alms houses with no medical facilities. Indeed the majority of the population had very little in the way of medical services, for the few physicians that existed were based in large towns and the remainder of the country had to depend on apothecaries, barber-surgeons, 'wise women' and - above all - self help.

In a predominantly rural community that was well-fed and healthy this was a tolerable situation. But the population had now enlarged and migrated into towns where both accommodation and working conditions were atrocious, and the problem of dealing with those who were sick and injured had become a matter of urgency. This was a challenge which, for various reasons, attracted the attention of three different groups. First and foremost were the philanthropists - many of them nonconformists - who added it to their existing concerns about housing, drunkenness, conditions at work, prisons, slavery and so on. Secondly there were the employers, not only of workers in industry but also of the army of domestic retainers on whose services polite society depended. Such people were of course anxious to get their employees back to work as soon as possible, but they also had the problem of what to do with them while they were ill. Finally there was the medical profession which, while by no means devoid of humanitarian sentiments, could also see a means of resolving this problem which was greatly to its advantage.

For all three groups the establishment of hospitals appeared to be the obvious solution. For patients and employers the advantages were apparent - the former had somewhere to go and the latter, who as subscribers acquired the right to refer patients to the hospital, had somewhere to send injured or ailing workmen and domestics.[1] For doctors - at least for those on the staff of the hospital - the benefits were more subtle but every bit as great. Such appointments enhanced the prestige of the incumbent and, in the course of soliciting funds for the institution, provided him with a legitimate excuse for making himself known to affluent members of the community. His income might be still further increased if such people sent their sons to him for training in the hope that, with the support of such an influential backer, they too would eventually obtain hospital appointments. Best of all, however, it allowed doctors to develop in medicine that spirit of enquiry which had already permeated other branches of learning, for it provided them with a group of 'captive' patients on whom new techniques could be tried out of sight of interfering relatives.

This attitude, relics of which still cause clashes between the profession and the public, was openly acknowledged. In the words of a 1767 textbook of surgery, 'hospitals funded by voluntary contributions have a direct tendency to promote and perfect knowledge of this art, making the benefit extend to all ranks of people'. (The extension was, of course, upwards!) A German professor was even more direct, pointing out that 'the hospital is not there to serve the patient, but the patient the hospital'. It was a point of view of which the general public was well aware although its response, understandably, varied. Speaking for the aristocracy one of George Eliot's characters observed that he 'had no objection if you like to try a few experiments on one of your hospital patients and kill a few people for charity. But I am not going to hand money out of my purse to have experiments tried on me'. The lower orders, understandably, saw matters in a somewhat different light and quickly decided that hospitals were 'schools of medicine where practitioners make experiments on the poor to improve themselves in the art of treating the rich'.

Hospitals, however, there had to be and in 1767 a group of local worthies, like their contemporaries in other English towns and cities, sat down to plan one for Leeds. Among the results of their deliberations there were two points of particular interest. The first was that the establishment was to be called The General Infirmary at Leeds - implying that it should be open to all and not (like the workhouse) exclusively for the residents of Leeds. The second was that, in contrast to medieval and continental hospitals, it was (to use the words of a contemporary manual) 'for the cure of the sick and not an alms-house for the support of the indigent and decrepit'. This meant that, as in many new hospitals, epileptics, lunatics and those who were pregnant, infectious, incurable or dying were not eligible for admission.

The first hospital was built on the site now occupied by the Yorkshire Bank in Infirmary Street, land which at that time was in open country beyond the salubrious west end of the town. It was, in the opinion of the philanthropist John Howard, 'one of the best hospitals in the kingdom' and one which even contrived to control infection, the great bane of such institutions, with the result that 'many are here cured of compound fractures who would lose their limbs in the unventilated and offensive wards of some older hospitals'. In general, however, it was unremarkable and despite a series of extensions which increased its capacity from 27 to 150 beds it eventually became evident that both it and the site were too small. In 1869 the Infirmary was therefore moved to its second (present) building, once more on the outskirts of the town behind the new Town Hall.

The new hospital, which had 300 beds, was destined to be a building of great architectural and scientific importance. Designed by George Gilbert Scott, who had just completed his most successful commission at St. Pancras Station, it bore a strong resemblance to that building both in its facade and in the great 'railway arch' which originally covered the central courtyard (Fig. 9). Similar too was the outstanding quality of the workmanship. This is immediately apparent in the great entrance hall, where each of the corbels supporting the roof timbers depicts a different plant used in medicine. But it extends throughout, reaching even the intricately carved stonework surrounding windows at the rear of the building which are barely visible to the public (Fig. 10).

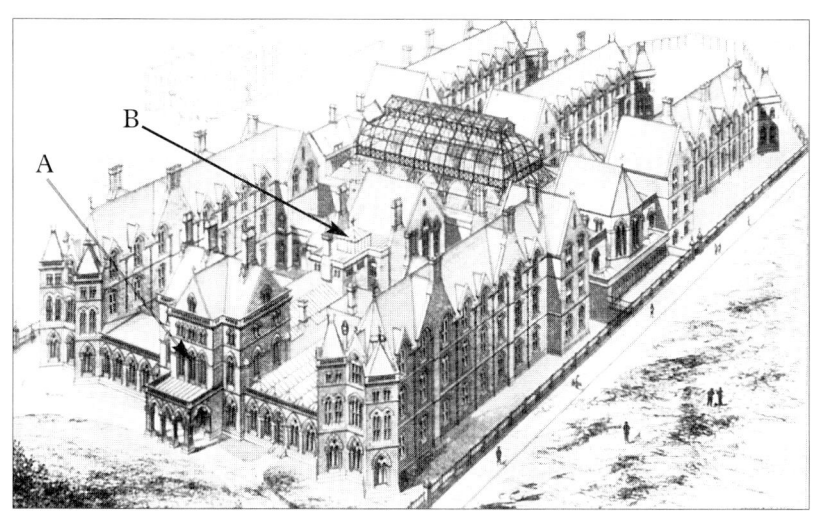

*Fig. 9. A bird's-eye view of the General Infirmary at Leeds, 1869. Note the separate ward blocks, the terminal 'claws' to contain the sluices and the 'railway arch' over the courtyard. The annual meeting room is marked (A) and the original operating theatre is marked (B).
(By kind permission of the Special Trustees of the Infirmary)*

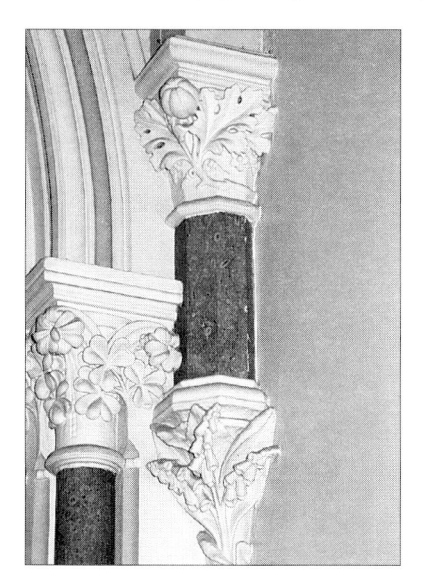

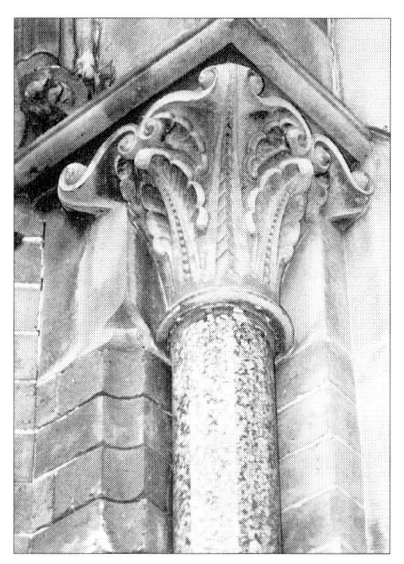

Fig. 10. One of the corbels depicting medicinal plants in the front hall, and stonework from an obscure window at the back of the hospital.

From a scientific point of view, however, the new Infirmary was of even greater importance. Hitherto most hospitals, like the houses of their wealthy patrons, had been built as solid blocks. Recent experience, particularly in the Crimean campaign, had however suggested that this was an unsatisfactory design because it provided insufficient ventilation. Other layouts had therefore been tried, as at St. Bartholomew's where James Gibbs' 1729 plan had set four separate ward blocks round a central square. Now, however, it was being suggested that in addition to having separate blocks no more than two stories high, wards should be designed with lofty ceilings and with windows facing both east and west. This was not an entirely new idea for a century earlier the French surgeon Tenon, sent by Louis XVI on a fact-finding mission, had reported favourably on the naval hospital at Plymouth that was built on this so-called pavilion plan. This, of course, had no immediate effect for France was about to be engulfed in the Revolution. But by 1862 a deputation from the Infirmary was able to visit a Parisian hospital - the Lariboisiere - built along these lines.

Even today, a visitor to this hospital can see at once how closely the design has been copied, for it too consists of a series of ward blocks ranged round an open courtyard that has a chapel at one end and a carriage arch at the other. The main difference is that, whereas the Lariboisiere is built on level ground, the Infirmary is built on a south-facing slope. To overcome this problem Scott 'wedged' an additional floor under the front of the building, so raising the two ward blocks on that side of the courtyard to the same level as the three at the back. The extra floor was used to house a sumptuous entrance, the entrance hall, the boardroom and the grand staircase. The only problem with this design is that, to this day, visitors who enter the rear of the building at ground level still wonder how they come to be on the first floor by the time they reach the front.

The immense success of this project was only marred by two things. In planning the building the committee had sought the advice of Florence Nightingale, whose influence is to be seen in the orientation and layout of the wards with their projecting terminal 'claws' that house well-ventilated sluices. Unfortunately Miss Nightingale's knowledge of finance proved to be less profound than her knowledge of hygiene, for in calculating the cost per bed of a *pavilion*-style hospital her estimate was wrong by a factor of four.

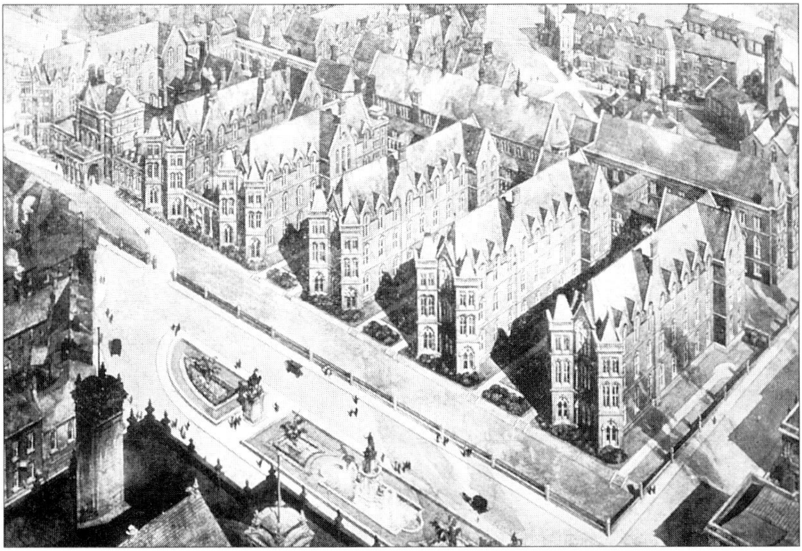

Fig. 11. A design, drawn up in 1910, which would have provided the General Infirmary at Leeds with six identical ward blocks along the south front. Sadly, it was rejected.
(By kind permission of the Special Trustees of the Infirmary)

An attempt to raise money by using the wards and galleries for a National Exhibition of Art and Design for six months before the hospital opened was also a failure. Despite the fact that it attracted over half a million visitors, it actually ran at a loss. The comments of the first patient who, when admitted with a fractured thigh, was presented with 'a Bible, suitably inscribed' are not recorded.

It would be nice to report that this fine building, once one of the most advanced hospitals in Europe, had been treated with respect. Sadly this has not been the case. The first extension - an additional (third) block of wards at the front - was entirely in keeping with the original design and in 1910 a far-seeing architect devised a scheme which would eventually have produced a frontage with six such matching bays (Fig. 11). Sadly this opportunity to produce a truly imposing building was rejected, with the result that Scott's elegant wards now stand alongside one block which has been likened to the back end of a passenger liner, a second which is nondescript[2] and a third that can only be described as a monstrosity. The area behind the hospital is, if anything, worse. In recent years plans for a fully integrated medical school and teaching hospital with nearly 1,300 beds floundered on a combination of altered specifications and government cutbacks. Instead a disintegrated hospital and medical school occupy a collection of large, un-coordinated and unlovely modern buildings. Yet amidst this clutter Scott's Infirmary, now 130 years old, remains intact, a landmark in the history of hospital design and a gem of Victorian architecture.

REFERENCES
Anning, S.T. The General Infirmary at Leeds. Livingstone, 1966.
Anning, S.T. The History of Medicine in Leeds. W.S.Maney and Son, 1980.

NOTES
1. In 1771 Edwin Lascelles, the future Baron Harewood - a generous benefactor who laid the foundation stone of the General Infirmary at Leeds - appointed his agent 'to recommend proper objects to your Infirmary in my name.' (Particularly in Yorkshire the term 'object' is used colloquially to describe 'a person of pitiable aspect.')
2. This extension is mainly notable for the fact that the eye department was given by the famous cricketer Prince Ranjitsinhji, who was treated at the Infirmary after a shooting accident in which he lost an eye. He continued to send a donation of 100 guineas each year on his birthday up to the time of his death.

CHAPTER XII

The Development of Surgery at Leeds

The building of the new Infirmary at Leeds coincided with the introduction of antiseptic surgery. The importance of this discovery is well illustrated by the rapid developments in theatre technique and theatres thereafter.

ONE OF THE oldest pictures in the Boardroom of The General Infirmary at Leeds shows **William Hey** (1736-1819), a founder-member of the staff, examining an injured peasant child under the watchful eyes of its surprisingly elegant 'mother'. Hey was renowned not only for his skill but also for his kindness to patients, a reputation which Lady Harewood decided to test by (rather unsuccessfully) assuming the guise of a country-woman and bringing the patient herself. So impressed was she by the results of her experiment that, so the story goes, she had this picture painted to record the event. Be that as it may, Hey, a Methodist who often entertained John Wesley in his house at No. 1 Albion Place (now the home of the Leeds' Law Society), was the first in the long line of distinguished surgeons for which the Infirmary is renowned. But the Infirmary is also interesting because it is still possible to trace in its buildings the rapid development of four separate operating theatres at the turn of the nineteenth century and to follow in its records the introduction of innovations which made these changes necessary.

Early surgery

When the new Infirmary was opened in 1869, surgeons were still the 'second class citizens' of medicine. Seven centuries earlier the Lateran Council had forbidden the clergy - who were largely responsible for the provision of medical services - to participate in any procedure that involved the shedding of blood and the College of Physicians had subsequently confirmed that it would have nothing to do with a demeaning craft of this sort. The Company of Barber Surgeons and the College of Surgeons were therefore left to their own devices. Yet despite these strictures the surgeons were in fact much better trained than the physicians, whose knowledge of physiology, methods of diagnosis and treatment were still rudimentary. From the time of Vesalius (1543) surgeons had had a sound knowledge of anatomy which they continued to improve through the wholesale dissection of stolen bodies. And while those centres of culture, the two great Universities, were still mulling over the works of Galen and the Arabist scholars - now more than 1,000 years old - schools of anatomy like the one run by the Hunters on the site of the Windmill Theatre in Soho were exploring the problems of physiology, pathology and obstetrics in a truly scientific manner.

Sadly this mine of information was of little practical value, for patients had to be in dire straits before they would face the unrelieved pain of an operation. By dint of working with great speed and precision the better surgeons did manage to obtain some remarkable results. Indeed in 1840 the Professor of Surgery at Amsterdam, unaware of the momentous events about to occur, observed that 'surgical art is at present within measurable distance of being perfect.' In point of fact the few operations done were virtually limited to the amputation of gangrenous or mangled limbs, 'cutting for the (bladder) stone', the couching of cataracts[1] and the occasional removal of a carcinomatous breast or an ovarian cyst so large that it was rendering the patient unsteady on her feet.

The introduction of anaesthesia in 1846 did little to improve the situation. Although it relieved the pain of the operation it was inherently dangerous, not least because it was left in the hands of a student or dresser who simply covered the patient's face with a towel onto which, at the direction of the surgeon, he poured generous quantities of chloroform. Apart from ensuring that he could still breathe he made no other observations.[2] Worse still, the technique tempted surgeons to undertake more complicated and dangerous procedures. But the main barrier to the practice of surgery was a new problem, hospital infections.

Septic surgery

With the development of hospitals and the concentration of patients in one place, post-operative infections had become common. Wards, according to contemporary observers, 'stank with the mawkish, manna-like odour of suppuration and not a single wound healed without festering'. The mortality from amputation, the most common procedure, was in the region of 50% and the anaesthetist Snow believed that 'a man laid on the operating table of one of our surgical hospitals is exposed to more chances of death than the English soldiers on the field of Waterloo.' Nor, under the circumstances, was this surprising, for at The London Hospital the theatre porter, who was also the post-mortem room attendant, described how surgeons wandered from one to the other without washing their hands. At Leeds the surgical staff operated as a group, 'putting their dirty fingers in any interesting wound and exhaling vapours from their sweaty dressing gowns'. Some wards had 'one sponge and basin to wash all wounds twice a day' and the idea of providing clean dressings for each patient (instead of having them rinsed and re-used) was regarded as extravagant. Such were the dangers that, in all seriousness, the surgeon Pirogoff said he would 'rather care for wounded soldiers in the most miserable of peasants' huts than in military hospitals'. Indeed, surgeons at the Infirmary *did* seek permission to carry out their operations elsewhere, and when the new Infirmary opened 20 years after the introduction of anaesthesia the average number of operations was still under one a day, a fifth of them being amputations.

For so small a workload one theatre was, of course, adequate, and it is still possible to trace the outline of this room, parts of which remain. It stood behind the double doors in the centre of the landing at the head of the main staircase - doors which are now the entrance to the Littlewood Hall. It was as wide as the first part of the lobby and extended through the facing wall to the far end of the office beyond. Illumination was provided by a strange horizontal window on the south side of that office, which still extends up into the roof, and by a lantern window over the lobby. This can be seen as a sort of glasshouse a little way behind the front entrance on the well-known bird's eye view of the hospital (Fig. 9). The patient, led directly into the theatre from the landing, would have found the floor covered with bloodstained sawdust and the air thick with smoke from the stove used to heat instruments for cautery.

There was no sink and instruments were kept on open shelves. Ranged round the room on tiered stands were the students, who entered the theatre via a spiral staircase from the front hall below, and in the foreground would be a group of surgeons in their theatre garb, 'old frock coats so impregnated with blood that they could be stood against the wall'. The wooden operating table was placed directly under the lantern window.

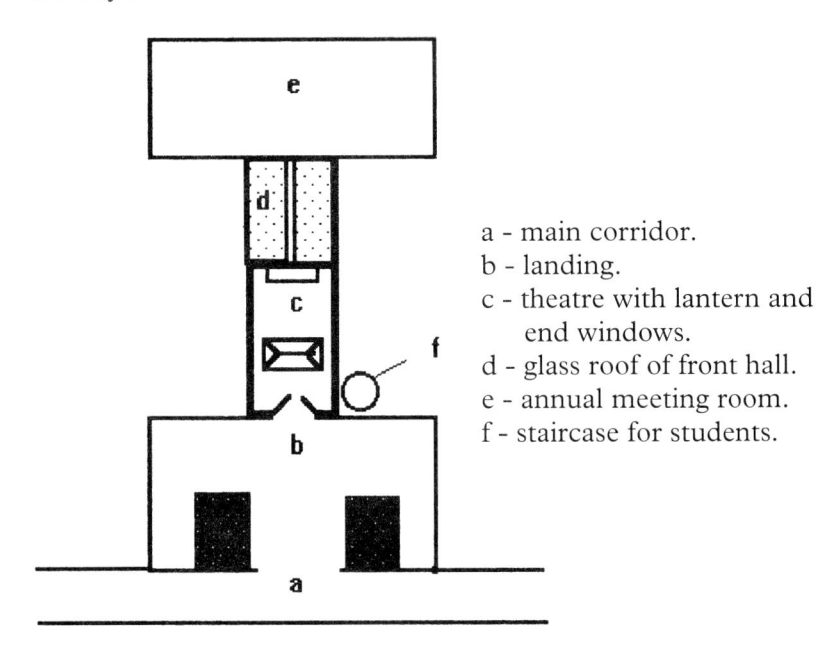

a - main corridor.
b - landing.
c - theatre with lantern and end windows.
d - glass roof of front hall.
e - annual meeting room.
f - staircase for students.

Antiseptic surgery

Theatres, however, were about to acquire a new piece of equipment, for in the year in which the new Infirmary opened Joseph Lister published his first paper on antiseptic surgery. Lister, like John Hunter, had been puzzled by the fact that whereas a compound fracture - one in which the broken bone is exposed through a skin wound - almost invariably became infected, a complicated fracture of the rib, in which the fractured ends pierced and were exposed to air in the lung, did not. The reason for this apparent paradox became evident when a colleague drew his attention to one of Pasteur's experiments which showed that if broth is stored in swan-neck containers - which protect it from dust but not from contact with the air - it does not putrefy. By a process of analogy this suggested that wound infections might be due, not to contact with air itself but to airborne micro-organisms which gained entry through the broken skin. Casting around for a means of preventing this, Lister recalled that in Carlisle the local refuse dumps were sprayed with carbolic acid to prevent putrefaction. He therefore devised a spray for use in theatre, a device which 'sent clouds of carbolic steam fizzing and spurting from large brass cylinders over everything.' He also arranged for dressings and ligatures to be soaked in carbolic acid and for ligatures to be cut short.[3]

The effect of these measures was astounding. Lister's patients were poor and malnourished and his wards and theatres were still filthy. Yet in the year following the introduction of the antiseptic technique many limbs were saved and the mortality among those who did require amputation fell from 45% to zero. It was an advance of which the Leeds surgeon Moynihan was to say 'nothing of which the world has knowledge has rescued so many lives.' Yet curiously it was an advance which the profession, at least in the United Kingdom, was slow to embrace, for when visiting the new Royal Infirmary at Edinburgh twelve years later Osler noted that 'Listerism is not making great headway even in this northern metropolis.' To some extent this was due to the innate conservatism of his colleagues, but there were also other reasons. For one thing carbolic acid had already been tried without success. Indeed according to Celsus it had been used in Ancient Rome, where wounds were treated with thymum, which contains a closely related chemical. Moreover, as the British Medical Journal pointed out in 1879, 'there is something, we will not say suspicious but at any rate strange in the persistent avoidance of the challenge thrown out to Mr. Lister and his followers to show, by actual comparison, whether and if so how far their results are really superior.' This strange reluctance to provide statistical evidence was eventually and effectively remedied by his registrar Watson Cheyne in a paper which, according to the same journal, 'revealed results so marvellous .... that they require no comment.'

The staff at the Infirmary evidently had mixed views about this new technique. Speaking in Leeds at the 1869 meeting of the British Medical Association Mr. Nunneley, who admitted that he had no personal experience of antiseptic surgery, said that his colleagues had used it for three years without obtaining results better than their own. This statement was immediately challenged by **Mr. Pridgin Teale** (1801-1867) who said that he and his fellow surgeons 'still used and had as much confidence as ever' in the new method. Records confirm that it was introduced early, in 1866, and that new sprays were ordered in 1879 and 1880. By 1874 the number of operations done at The General Infirmary at Leeds had doubled and between 1875 and 1890 removals of ovarian cysts (virtually the only operation attempted on the abdomen) increased four-fold in number with a coincidental fall in mortality from 73% to 15%.

These developments had a profound effect on the status of surgeons who, from being second class citizens, suddenly emerged as the only people who had an effective treatment to offer. Able at last to utilise their knowledge of anatomy they quickly extended their repertoire and assumed pride of place in the hierarchy of the hospital. The development also resulted in a demand for more theatre space and in 1885, less than twenty years after the Infirmary was built, the first extensions appeared on either side of the old theatre. Double doors were installed at the heads of the staircases on either side. Those on the east led into a lobby which in turn led into an anaesthetic room on the left, a new, smaller theatre in front and the old theatre on the right. The doors at the head of the west staircase led to a room known until recently as the surgeons' room, and beyond this there was a room for students.

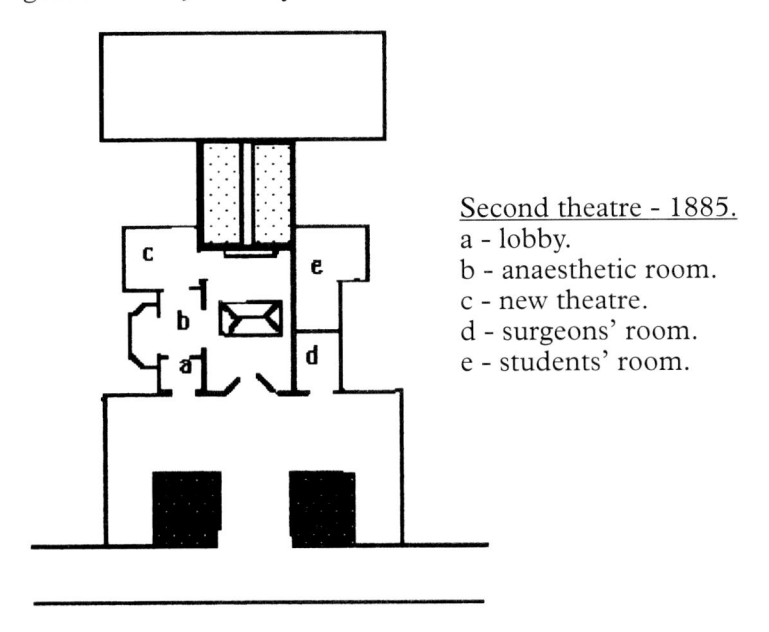

Second theatre - 1885.
a - lobby.
b - anaesthetic room.
c - new theatre.
d - surgeons' room.
e - students' room.

Aseptic surgery

The antiseptic spray was not, however, the final solution. This cumbersome device had been designed to kill the airborne bacteria supposedly responsible for wound infection. But by the mid 1880s Lister came to realise that most infections stemmed, not from the air but from fingers and instruments that came into contact with the wound. The spray was therefore abandoned, and Cushing was astounded to find a senior officer of the Royal College of Surgeons still using one (to the consternation of his junior staff) in 1900.[4] Instead, emphasis was placed on the sterilisation of instruments and on Treves' doctrine that 'the secret of surgery is in the nailbrush.' As always, however, it was an uphill battle and in 1899 the British Medical Journal, reacting to criticism of conditions in London operating theatres, still found it impossible to believe 'in the high septicity of an English gentleman's fingernails.'

This, however, was not the only development in theatre technique for in 1896, when the Infirmary obtained 'two fish kettles for sterilising instruments, to be heated by electricity' it also provided 'linen coats for any of the operating staff who wish to use them.' This presumably was at the behest of a newly appointed assistant surgeon called Moynihan, for whom the old frock coats worn by his seniors were not good enough. Seven years later he returned from America with an even more remarkable innovation - rubber gloves, which had been introduced by Halsted for the benefit of a theatre sister (later his wife) who had developed contact dermatitis. The students thought that this was hilarious and in the 1903 Christmas revue warned the nurses that

We see the surgeons turn aside, to test the latest germicide,
To stop the wily microbe's least infection;
They've sterile clothes from top to toe - moustaches now have had
   to go,
And even just to speak will bring correction.
But not content their hair to hide, when on the nurses fair they've
   spied,
They'll order caps too hideous to mention.
Lest when they're on a mighty list, *their* doings may be slightly
   missed,
And *you* should claim the gallery's attention.
There's no doubt it must impress to thus cover up each tress,
But I think it's cutting things a bit too fine ... ah.

For quite soon they'll want to veil every face from gaze of male,
You'd be better far in convents out in China.

Their predictions were, of course, absolutely correct - the only thing they failed to foresee was Moynihan's theatre boots at which a visiting French surgeon gazed in amazement, asking 'Does he stand *in* the abdomen?'

The increasing complexity of the procedures and the rising volume of work meant that in 1897 - a mere twelve years after the previous modification - the theatres had to be enlarged for a second time. On this occasion two identical suites were provided, one on each side of the original theatre. Waiting rooms were built behind the doors at the heads of the east and west staircases, each of which led to anaesthetic rooms (now lavatories). These in turn led to the theatres (now a student's room on the east and a seminar room on the west) the roof-lights of which can still be seen from the outside. The fate of the large windows in the south walls will be mentioned later. The old theatre was partitioned as it is now, the front (office) half becoming a room in which instruments were stored and sterilised and the back half a lobby which contained a recovery room and a surgeons' room on either side of the exit through the central

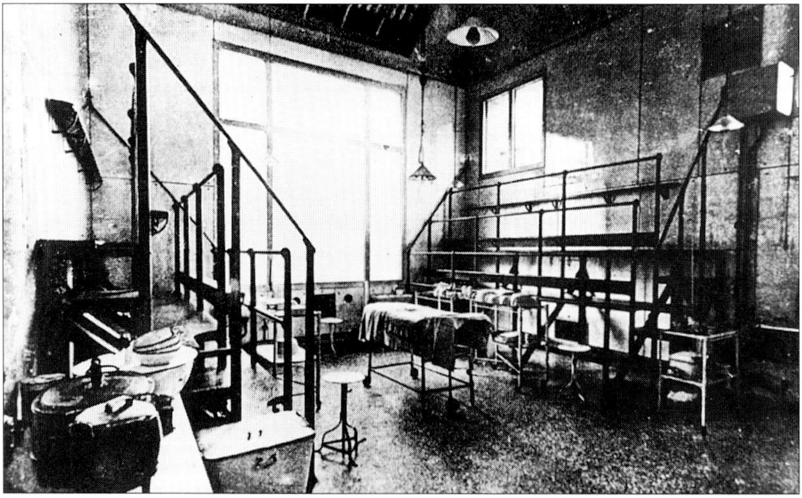

Fig. 12. One of the twin theatres in the General Infirmary at Leeds, built in 1897. Note the large south window and the roof light above.
(By kind permission of the Special Trustees of the Infirmary)

doors. This suite, while younger than the famous building at Guy's, retains far more of its original features and must be among the oldest operating theatres in the country.

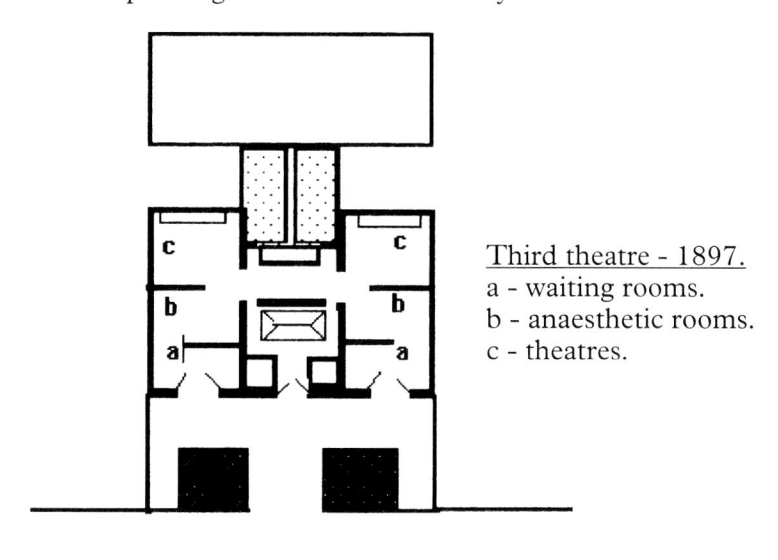

Third theatre - 1897.
a - waiting rooms.
b - anaesthetic rooms.
c - theatres.

Following the completion of these new theatres the remorseless rise in the amount of surgical activity continued and within twenty years a further enlargement, the fourth since the opening of the hospital fifty years earlier, had to be undertaken. The fact that this new development was to serve the hospital for more than fifty years gives some indication of the speed with which surgery grew at the end of the 19th century. These theatres, however, were on a new site and the original theatre, along with its extensions, was to become part of a teaching block named after **Harry Littlewood** (1861-1921) the first Professor of Surgery at the University of Leeds.

From theatre to lecture hall

The Littlewood Hall development incorporated another interesting room which can be seen above the front porch on old prints of the hospital (Fig. 9). Originally isolated from the rest of the building, this Annual Meeting Room could only be reached via a flight of stairs behind the porters' lodge. Sadly there does not appear to be a picture of it, but from its commanding position, its huge fireplace and a fragment of the original plaster ceiling which survives just behind the front windows it seems to have been imposing. This, of course, is hardly surprising, for its main function was to house the annual meeting of the patrons of the hospital - an event of some importance, for in addition to their donations this group was responsible for the election of the consultant staff. This arrangement, as might be expected, ensured that virtually all consultants came from the locality, often from families which had produced several consultants and even several generations of consultants.[5] Elections were keenly contested and canvassing, far from being forbidden, was essential. Candidates, moreover, were expected to provide transport for their supporters - an expensive exercise which, in 1835, cost one Manchester surgeon £700. Other less reputable ploys included the bribing of opponents and, in an election in Leeds in 1864, the circulation of letters which even the Lancet deemed too libellous to publish. The appointment of a new

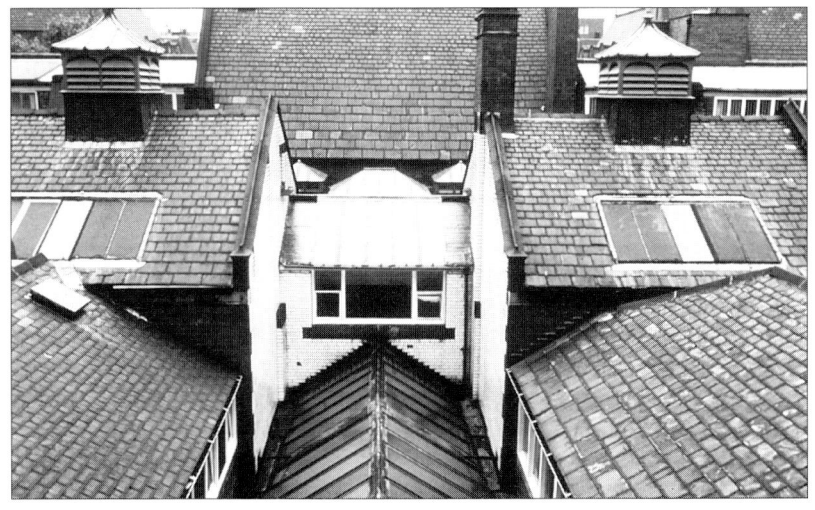

Fig. 13. A view of the old theatre block at the General Infirmary at Leeds as seen looking backwards from above the main entrance. The pale building in the centre is the original theatre, visible on fig. 9, and the lantern window can be seen beyond. On either side are the twin theatres of 1897 with the roof lights intact. The south windows of these theatres have been obliterated by extensions that run backwards on either side of the glass roof over the front hall.

consultant was therefore a matter which aroused considerable public interest, and despite the fact that ladies voted by proxy such events had been known to attract nearly 500 delegates, forcing the meeting to adjourn to a more commodious venue.

The use of so elegant a room was, of course, strictly limited and apart from examinations and lectures the other main events which it accommodated were the lectures of the Leeds and West Riding Medico-Chirurgical Society. Founded in 1872 this society, the oldest medical society in Leeds, was responsible for an extension built onto the north-west corner of the annual meeting room. This is marked on the 1895 plans as the microscope room, which gives some indication of the belated interest in medical microscopy occasioned by the development of bacteriology and histology at the end of the nineteenth century. More importantly, however, this room was the first stage in the development of two extensions which, by 1928, ran on either side of the glass roof of the hall to link the annual meeting room with the main building via the south windows of the twin operating theatres (Fig. 13). The extension on the west was to become the Garland Gallery, named after **Hugh Garland**, the first neurologist at the Infirmary. The extension on the east is an office corridor leading into the annual meeting room which in 1968 (after being used for lectures and examinations), was converted into the Littlewood Hall.

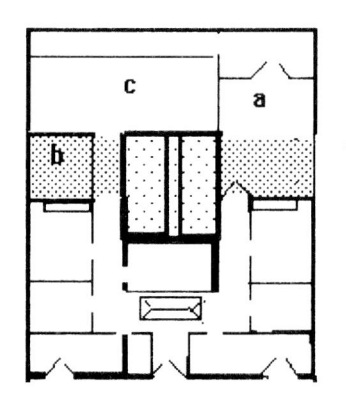

The Littlewood Hall Suite - 1928.
a - Garland Gallery.
b - extension from east theatre.
c - annual meeting room/
   Littlewood Hall.

Set within the teaching block, however, the structure of the operating theatres which served the Infirmary from its inception and which witnessed the development of modern surgery is still clearly visible. Standing under the lantern window in the lobby, the visitor is on the site occupied by the operating table in the days when antiseptic surgery was in its infancy. It was here that **Thomas Jessop** (1837-1903) removed the first Wilm's tumour of the kidney in 1877 and where **Andrew Fergusson McGill** (1846-1890) did the first suprapubic prostatectomy ten years later. Moving a little to left or right, he enters the theatres where **Sir Arthur Mayo-Robson** (1853-1933; Front cover) pioneered the surgery of the gall bladder and bile ducts and **Lord Moynihan** (1865-1936), the first (and still virtually the only) provincial President of the Royal College of Surgeons operated. Few hospitals have theatre blocks of such antiquity or have been served by such venerable surgeons - men who are remembered to this day by the names of the instruments which they designed.

REFERENCES
Anning, S.T. The General Infirmary at Leeds. Livingstone 1966.
Parsons, M. The old operating theatres of The General Infirmary at Leeds. Yorkshire Medicine, Winter 1993 10.

NOTES
1. ie pushing the opaque lens out of the line of vision.
2. The 'ether' or anaesthetic chart - regarded by some as America's greatest contribution to surgery - was invented by Harvey Cushing in 1895 after a patient he was required to anaesthetise while yet a student died.
3. Hitherto the long ends of unsterilised ligatures had been left protruding from the wound. Apart from being a potent source of infection the removal of these ligatures, by pulling them out some time after the operation, often resulted in a catastrophic haemorrhage.
4. **Geoffrey Wooler**, the first thoracic surgeon at Leeds, recalls that as late as 1930 the main theatre at The London Hospital still contained large tanks marked Acid Carbol. in the dilutions recommended by Lister.
5. In London, for example, the surgeon Astley Cooper had no less than five relatives on the staff of his hospital, one of whom was bitterly attacked for his incompetence by Thomas Wakley in his journal The Lancet (at that time the 'Private Eye' of medicine). Wakley, not having the right contacts, had been unable to obtain an appointment.

CHAPTER XIII

Clifford Allbutt and the Development of Modern Medicine

At a time when 'doing the tests' threatens the traditional methods of interrogation and examination it is interesting to look back on the introduction of investigations.

'WE', REPLIED OSLER, when asked how he and his companion should be announced, 'Are the brothers Regii'. It was a clever answer, for the parallels between Sir William, Regius Professor of Physic at Oxford and Sir **Thomas Clifford Allbutt** (1836-1925), Regius Professor at Cambridge, were remarkable. Both were the sons of clergymen; both were distinguished physicians; both had produced famous textbooks of medicine; both, exhausted by clinical duties, had accepted academic posts; both received the Fellowship of the Royal College of Physicians in the same year; and both, incredibly, had given the Goulstonian Lecture at the College. This last at least should have been impossible, for that lecture is traditionally given by one of the four most junior Fellows. But in 1883, the year of Allbutt's oration, no Fellowships had been conferred. This came about because one of those proposed was a physician at a hospital which accepted female students and the President, a confirmed misogynist, had refused to accept the nomination. The governing body promptly retaliated by rejecting all the other candidates, leaving the College without any new Fellows and therefore without a lecturer for the following year. They therefore had to nominate a second speaker from Allbutt's year - William Osler.

There was, however, one important difference, for Osler was a Canadian. Allbutt, by contrast, was a Yorkshireman, a son of the vicar of Dewsbury who had been educated at St. Peter's in York.[1]

For some time he had been uncertain about his future career, for he had many talents. He had a sound knowledge of English and Classical literature and was friendly with Hardy, the Brontes and George Eliot. He was an artist and a musician, being involved, among other things, in the purchase of the famous Schulze organ bought by a neighbour for his wife and installed in a vast extension to their house in Meanwood.[2] But he also had a great interest in science and in the long run it was this, along with his contacts with other doctors in the family, that caused him to opt for medicine. He qualified at St. George's Hospital in 1861 and, after working for a time with Trousseau and Duchenne in Paris, joined the staff of The General Infirmary at Leeds in 1864.

Allbutt could hardly have chosen a more propitious time or place to enter the profession. After stagnating for nearly 2,000 years the face of medicine had been transformed by that unsung triumph of the French Revolution, the Medical School of Paris. Physicians who, until recently, had dispensed advice from the comfort of a coffee house were now using the techniques of palpation, percussion and auscultation it had introduced to examine their patients. Physical signs were being carefully compared with autopsy findings and, by degrees, a picture of different diseases each with its own symptoms, signs and pathology was emerging. The process, however, was far from complete and for a young doctor, inspired by his experiences in Paris and about to enter one of the most modern hospitals in Europe, the opportunities were immense.

To modern eyes, Allbutt's contributions seem at first to be fairly mundane. It must, however, be remembered that the development of British hospital medicine had only just begun and that for his contemporaries his ideas, all of which have stood the test of time, were of considerable significance. Indeed to older readers the abolition of one of his reforms - the hospital trained nurse - has been one of the greatest disasters to hit modern medicine. Two years after he was appointed Allbutt complained that the 'nurses' in the Infirmary were required to scrub the floors. The nurses of the time were, however, 'great powerful red-faced women who all ate a great deal of beef and drank a great deal of beer and lifted patients as you would lift puppy-dogs'. Allbutt was aware that Miss Nightingale, fresh from her triumphs in the Crimea, had started a school for nurses of a very different sort at St. Thomas's Hospital and by 1866 steps were being taken to establish a similar school at Leeds.

Allbutts' interests in clinical medicine were many and varied. He was, for example, an early advocate of the prevention of deep venous thrombosis and of the open air treatment of fevers - a regime he is said to have adopted because it had been noticed that Irish peasants abandoned at the roadside fared better than those admitted to hospital. He advocated the use of morphia for 'cardiac asthma' and the tapping of pericardial and pleural effusions (a technique he had learned from Trousseau) - ideas which, in an institution in which the senior physician still thought that the surgeons should be brought in to give injections, were highly controversial! But more importantly, he was associated with the introduction of five pieces of equipment that have been in use ever since. In talking of these developments it must again be remembered that in 1860 the idea of *examining* a patient, imported from France, was still relatively new. Mechanical aids to diagnosis, apart from a stethoscope and a pocket watch with a second hand (introduced at the turn of the century)[3] did not exist. Allbutt's first simple request (made in 1866), for a machine with which to weigh patients, was therefore - at that stage - a novelty.

At much the same time Allbutt was involved in the development of the clinical thermometer. Thermometers and even small thermometers had been available since the 17th century, but those currently in clinical use had to be kept in position for 25 minutes and read in situ. They were therefore about a foot long and crook-shaped (Fig. 14). As might be expected, these cumbersome

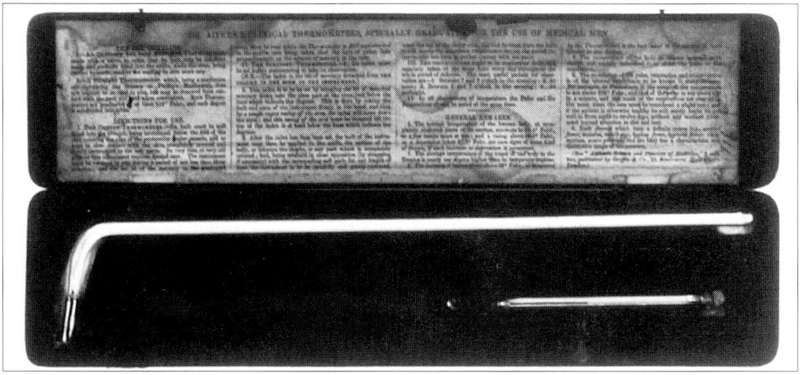

Fig. 14. Allbutt's thermometer and the crook-shaped thermometer it replaced. (By kind permission of the Special Trustees of the Infirmary)

instruments were only used by a few enthusiasts. After a series of experiments, however, Allbutt contrived to design one that was only six inches long. It took five minutes to record the temperature and later versions had the familiar constriction beyond the bulb so that it could be removed and read at leisure. Early versions were not, however, popular because of his insistence that they should be graduated in Centigrade. Once this was replaced by the more familiar Fahrenheit scale they quickly became (and remained) an essential item of medical equipment.[4]

Allbutt's third aid to clinical examination was based on his belief that, having answered the questions 'what is disease?' and 'where is disease?' the time had come to ask 'why is disease?' In other words he thought that examining the end results of an illness at autopsy, although interesting as an exercise, was of limited practical value. If lethal cerebral haemorrhages, for example, were to be *prevented* the 'mine' of hypertension had to be detected before it exploded. This, at a time when sphygomanometers did not exist, was a very advanced idea, yet by 1870 Allbutt was trying to record the blood pressure.[5] Soon after he was suggesting that everyone over the age of 40 should have their blood pressure checked every five years so that the onset of essential hypertension could be observed - a recommendation, yet to be implemented, which has stood the test of time. The treatment he suggested - mountaineering - has not!

The fourth aid to diagnosis pioneered by Allbutt - ophthalmoscopy - was a more sophisticated technique. Introduced by Helmholtz in 1850[6] it was promoted in England by the ophthalmologist and ovariotomist **Spencer Wells**, a Leeds student. Initially the idea was greeted with enthusiasm, for the ability to examine what was in effect part of the brain - the tip of the optic nerve - promised to be of great value in the diagnosis of neurological disorders. But due to technical difficulties and lack of information about the appearance of the normal, let alone the abnormal retina it was soon abandoned by the majority.

Allbutt, however, had the good fortune to work with two people who were not so easily discouraged. As a student at St. George's Hospital he encountered John Ogle, a pathologist who argued that as there was a close relationship between the retinal and cerebral circulations the former might well provide information about the latter. During his postgraduate studies in Paris he also encountered Duchenne, another early advocate of ophthalmoscopy. On returning to Leeds he therefore made a careful study of the fundi, not only of his own patients but also of selected patients in the asylums at Wakefield and at Clifton in York. As the first person to describe the histological changes in the cerebral arteries of patients with syphilis he was disappointed to find that they were not reflected, as Ogle had predicted, in the retina. But he accumulated a wealth of information about the appearance of the healthy fundus and the characteristic changes found in patients with cerebral tumours, general paralysis of the insane, renal disease, tuberculous meningitis and other disorders. Initially presented in a series of papers and lectures this information was eventually brought together in 1871 in a book entitled *On the use of the ophthalmoscope in diseases of the nervous system and of the kidneys; also in certain other general disorders*. Written at a time 'when you could count on the fingers of one hand the physicians who were using it' this was the first English treatise on ophthalmoscopy. It did not revolutionise practice, for during the first World War Cushing was still complaining that he was the only person in the hospital who knew how to use an ophthalmoscope. But with the work of Hughlings Jackson (to whom the book was dedicated) and Gowers it did rescue from oblivion what was to become one of the most important components of the clinical examination.

Allbutts final contribution to scientific medicine, at least in Leeds, was the promotion of microscopy. To present-day readers, for whom the two are inextricably linked, it must seem incredible that the microscope was ignored and even derided by the profession until a little over a century ago. First introduced at the start of the 17th century it was still being denigrated at the start of the 19th - 'the kind of agent from which physiology and anatomy never appear to derive much help because looking at things in the dark makes everyone see them in his own way'. By the middle of the century (when the anthrax bacillus had been seen) attitudes were starting to change and it was even admitted that the instrument 'might replace hypothesis with evidence'. In that it led to the development of cellular pathology and the revolutionary discoveries of bacteriology this was, if anything, an understatement. Allbutt was therefore well to the fore in requesting a microscope for the Infirmary in 1869, for twenty years later the University of Pennsylvania still had only one such instrument

Allbutt's contributions to the technology of medicine must not however be allowed to give the impression that he was a hospital-based boffin. On the contrary, he was a highly respected clinician whose services were much in demand from the Trent to the Tees. His income was substantial and he was able to build a magnificent home for his family at Carr Manor to the north of Leeds, where his initials can still be seen in the wrought iron gates.[7] In addition, he managed to participate in the wider aspects of his profession, joining in debates about the organisation of medicine, becoming an authority on its history and - in a measure which has only recently become generalised - persuading his colleagues in Leeds to agree medical evidence before appearing in court.

The strain of this work was, however, becoming unbearable and in 1889, to the surprise of his colleagues, he abandoned clinical practice and moved to London where he became a Commissioner in Lunacy. Through his contacts with the West Riding Lunatic Asylum he had a long-standing interest in mental illness and it is perhaps unfortunate that he did not persist with this work. In 1892, however, he moved yet again, this time to become the Regius Professor of Physic at Cambridge.

If the University thought it was appointing a professor whose first interest was in clinical medicine it was to be sorely disappointed. From the outset Allbutt made plain his opinion that 'any opportunities for gaining professional knowledge here are adventitious and might even become means of danger did we not always bear in mind that the chief function of a university must be to promote a harmonious development of all the faculties of man.' Clearly Cambridge was falling short of this objective, for looking at the contemporary medical student he 'observed to my pain that he is by no means learned; that too often he thinks loosely and that he does not always write even the English of the gentlemen who do the Fires and the Murders for country journals. On his Latinity I will keep a discrete silence.' His efforts to remedy this situation aroused considerable interest. He decided that the best way to make students think and to test this ability was to introduce a thesis into the MB examination. To ensure that this was properly written he also issued for his students *Notes on the Composition of Scientific Papers* 'to save his time and theirs in clerical revision of theses'. On discovering that some at least of these papers were the work of 'ghost' writers he simply asked the candidates to read out their offerings and discuss such parts as the examiner chose.

Needless to say these activities did not go unnoticed in the university, and the Cambridge Review gleefully reported

There's an awful row in Cambridge and its starter is no lesser
Than a most important person who is likewise a Professor;
For he said 'The reason Cambridge fails, while Oxford's
   a success is   – Essays'.

If we only were like Oxford we might safely hope to win
Situations on some journals which as yet won't let us in;
And the key that will unlock for us the portal to the Press is
                                                         – Essays.

So memorialists by the dozens drew a letter up to state
'Our facility in English is at best inadequate;
And the cure we would assure you for our obvious distress is
                                                         – Essays'

Then the Special Boards are summoned to discuss the situation;
They admit we are a failure without any hesitation;
'There's one only panacea' - every Special Board confesses
                                                         – Essays.

So hurrah! for the Professor who has shown us our sterility,
For we soon shall be possessors of an adequate facility,
For we're adding to the number of our pre-existing messes
                                                         – Essays.

    One wonders what Allbutt would have made of a world in which even senior qualifications can be obtained by putting ticks in squares!

    Sadly, in other respects his reception at Cambridge was less happy, for his colleagues at Addenbrooke's refused for a long time to provide him with any beds. This, however, he turned to advantage by editing his vast *System of Medicine* which was for many years a standard work of reference. He also displayed his versatility, his literary skills and his sense of humour by producing a *System of Gynaecology* for, as he pointed out, one had to sympathise with the patient 'entangled in the web of the gynaecologist who finds that her uterus, like her nose, is a little on one side, or again like that organ is running a little, or is as flabby as her biceps so that the unhappy organ is impaled on a stem, or perched on a prop, or is painted with carbolic acid every week in the year except during the vacation when the gynaecologist is grouse shooting, or salmon-catching, or leading the fashion in the Upper Engadine.' Medicine may have become more scientific, but it is a lot less entertaining.

REFERENCES

Miller, H. Two great contemporaries. World Medicine, October 9th, 1974, 15.

Rolleston, H. Life of Clifford Allbutt. Macmillan 1929.

NOTES

1. One of the oldest schools in the country, the fore-runner of which once had on its staff Alcuin, Charlemagne's adviser.
2. This magnificent instrument is now in St. Bartholomew's Church, Armley.
3. The ancient Egyptians knew how to compare the rate of the patient's pulse with the doctor's and in the 4th century BC Herophilus used a water clock to time the heart. Galen also observed a female patient with a mysterious illness who developed tachycardia when the name of a well-known actor was mentioned.
4. Allbutt, who was a keen mountaineer, used one of these instruments to record his own temperature while climbing. He also left an interesting account of the way in which the ability to speak languages learned later in life is lost (as in old age) while ascending a mountain without oxygen.
5. The blood pressure was first recorded (in animals) in 1733 by the Rev. Stephen Hales, using an arterial cannula and a glass tube 11 feet in length. He also devised a 'tonometer', an instrument with which others experimented in the early part of the 19th century. Cushing discovered the Riva Rocci device for measuring blood pressure when he toured Europe after his brief visit to the Infirmary in 1900 and took it back to America to add to his 'ether (anaesthetic) chart'. He seems to have been unaware that Allbutt had been working in this field for 30 years.

6. The escapologist Houdini also devised a method of examining his own retina.
7. The estate was subsequently bought by Lord Moynihan and one interesting relic - now in a patch of land sold for housing - is 'Moynihan's pond', which once contained a rare species of sinistral snails (snails with shells which curled in the reverse of the usual direction). These unfortunately were accidentally poisoned during the second world war, but records of them are held by the Leeds Museum (Fig. 15).

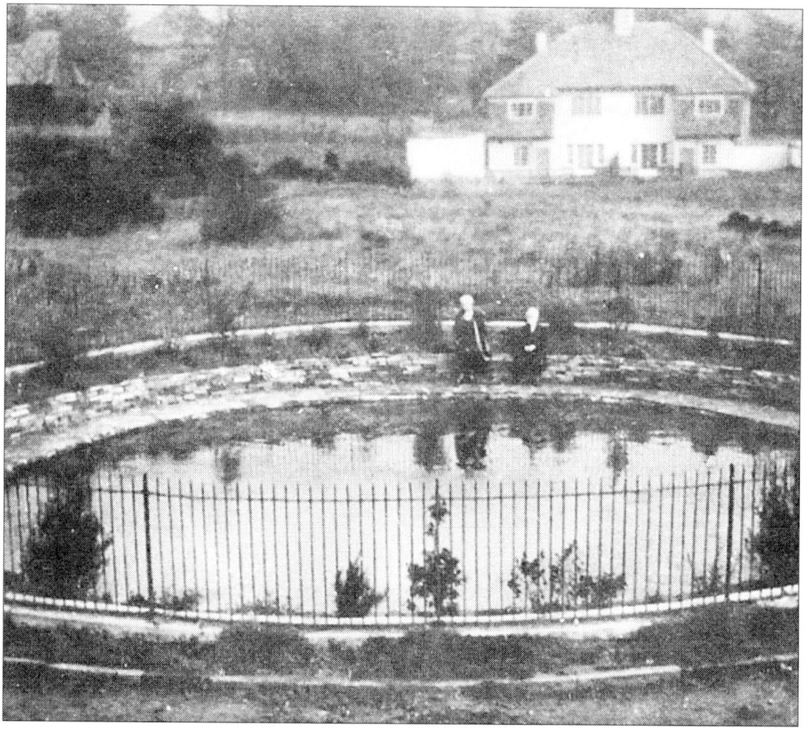

Fig. 15. 'Moynihan's pond', originally part of the Carr Manor estate he bought from Clifford Allbutt and now preserved in Southlands Drive, Leeds. (By kind permission of The Leeds Weekly News)

CHAPTER XIV

The Lessons of History

IN CONCLUSION, IT is interesting to consider the present state of medicine in the light of this story. The medicine practised by Clifford Allbutt, although undoubtedly 'modern', was in fact rudimentary. But whereas the doctors and hospitals of Allbutt's time were venerated their successors, although infinitely more accomplished, are widely criticised. This criticism comes not only from a vociferous minority whose complaints are fostered by the media, but also from a silent majority which is clearly deeply dissatisfied with the present service. In essence, their complaints seem to be based on the loss of four things.

The first is sanctuary - a bed, simple but dignified care and the relief of pain (sometimes provided by a cottage hospital), and the 'asylum' which allows those whose minds are disturbed to escape from the worries of the world. Needed as much now as they were when they were provided by monastic foundations or the philanthropists of the eighteenth and nineteenth centuries, they cannot be replaced by 'proper' hospitals where the cost of technology has so reduced the number of beds that they are in a permanent state of crisis.

The second is the unfashionable virtue of sacrifice. The hospital trained nurse who replaced the *religious* retained not only the title of sister but also, in effect, her vows of chastity, for until recently most ward sisters were unmarried. Some even lived in flats adjacent to their wards,[1] providing a level of care and supervision which, by today's standards, defies imagination. The same, indeed, applied to the nursing staff, for as recently as 1966 the historian of the Infirmary, **S.T. Anning**, wrote that a trainee 'might hope to become a staff nurse if she did not give up her career to get married.' Tyrannical though some of these ladies were, their meticulous care of patients and their vast experience of medicine were the very backbone of the hospital service. They also provided the highly regulated environment in which modern medicine was able to develop.

By the same token, although with little in the way of altruistic motives, every newly qualified doctor spent at least a year in hospital, more or less permanently on duty. This system was designed primarily to provide the incumbent with experience after his long academic training and to ensure the smooth running of the unit, for at this stage the houseman's knowledge of practical medicine was limited. Nevertheless, the collective experience of the 'doctors' mess' combined with that of the (apprentice trained) nursing staff was formidable. But above all, patients were reassured by the fact that 'their' doctor, who had at least a fundamental knowledge of their problems, was always available.

The third, and in many ways the most alarming failure of modern hospitals, is the decline in service. Thirty years ago the smallest unit could at least guarantee rest, quiet and exemplary personal care. The modern ward, by contrast, it is all too often a scene of squalid turmoil in which beds are unmade, patients are unwashed, and drugs are forgotten. The reappearance of bedsores and of 'hospital sepsis' are particularly alarming. One cannot but notice that this decline started when the ward sister was replaced by the 'nursing officer' and apprentice-style training by 'Nursing 2,000'.

The fourth and final need is for authority. The medical profession has been much criticised for its 'god-like attitude', and one objective of the introduction of management was to reduce doctors to the level of all other employees. But hospitals were founded at the instigation of doctors so that their patients could receive certain forms of treatment and they alone - if they are honest and courageous enough so to do - can ask the right questions and make the correct demands. Can the junior staff provide adequate cover and receive adequate training if they only work one night in five? Has the cost of technology so eroded the number of beds that basic services can no longer be provided? Is modern nursing delivering the care and attention patients require? Indeed, to what extent has the introduction of the new 'academic' form of nursing been responsible for the lack of recruits and the difficulty in retaining staff? These are hard questions which run counter to social and professional aspirations and even to the rule of law. But if sanctuary and service are to be restored, sacrifice has to be made for, as Enoch Powell so memorably observed, 'Hospitals should be run for the benefit of patients and not for the benefit of those working in them.'

Authority, service, sacrifice, sanctuary - they are not words which one associates with modern medicine. But they were the very basis of the religious foundations which, nearly 2,000 years ago, created the first hospitals. They did so in response to a command which still adorns the wall of the Medical School at Leeds - AEGROTOS SANATE, LEPROSOS PURGATE; DONO ACCEPISTIS, DONO DATE. (Heal the sick, cleanse the lepers, ... freely have ye received, freely give.) Is it this ancient lesson that we have forgotten?

NOTES
1. A colleague recalls how, on certain nights, the curtains round the beds were drawn as sister processed down the ward from her rooms to take her bath.

Glossary

Aesculapia - temples of the Greek god of healing, Aesculapius.

Aphasia - impairment of speech due to damage to the cortex of the brain.

Ascites - an accumulation of fluid in the abdomen.

Auscultation - listening to the sound of the heart or of air entering the lungs.

Autopsy - a post-mortem examination.

Bornholm disease - epidemic pain in the chest.

Cardiac asthma - bouts of breathlessness due to heart failure.

Cerebral hemispheres - the paired masses that form the main part of the brain.

Chorea - involuntary 'dancing' - ie twitching - movements.

Contact dermatitis - a skin rash caused by exposure to a substance to which the patient is sensitive.

Cord - the spinal cord - the mass of nervous tissue linking the brain with the peripheral nerves.

Corpora quadrigemina - a structure on the back of the lower part of the brain.

Cortex - the cerebral cortex - the wrinkled outer part of the cerebral hemispheres.

Cupping - the application of heated cups to the skin to 'bleed' the patient by drawing away blood.

Decussation - crossing from one side of the brain to the other.

Deep venous thrombosis - formation of a clot in the veins of the leg.

Epithelioma - a cancer of the skin.

Euthanasia - 'mercy-killing'.

Faradism - stimulation with a rapidly alternating electric current.
Fibrosis - scarring.
Focal fits - fits confined to, or starting in, one part of the body.
Frontal lobes - the front part of the cerebral hemispheres.
Fundus - the back of the eye, seen through the pupil.
Galvanism - stimulation with a uni-directional current.
General paralysis of the insane (G.P.I.) - syphilitic infection of the substance of the brain.
Glioma - a malignant tumour of the brain.
Hemiparesis - weakness of one side of the body.
Humour - one of the four fluids (blood, phlegm, yellow and black bile) whose balance was believed to determine personality and whose imbalance was thought to cause disease.
Hydrotherapy - treatment by immersion in water.
Hypertension - high blood pressure.
Interstitial keratitis - inflammation of part of the eye.
Labyrinthitis - a disturbance of the organ of balance.
Malignant - cancerous.
Motor cortex - the part of the cerebral cortex that controls movement.
Motor end-plate - the structure that links a motor nerve to the muscle.
Motor nerves - the nerves which control movement.
Obstetrics - the medicine of pregnancy and childbirth
Ophthalmoscope - instrument used to illuminate and examine the back of the eye.
Orbits - the recesses in the skull in which the eyes lie.
Ovariotomy - the removal of an ovarian tumour.
Pathology - the study of diseased tissues or organs.
Percussion - tapping the chest to detect areas of abnormal resonance which indicate disease.
Pericardial effusion - an abnormal collection of fluid in the space around the heart.
Physiology - the study of how the organs of the body work.

Pleural effusion - an abnormal collection of fluid in the chest around the lungs.

Relapsing fever - a disease transmitted by lice that causes intermittent bouts of fever.

Retina - the light-sensitive membrane at the back of the eye.

Scrotum - the pouch which contains the testes.

Sphygmomanometer - a machine used to measure the blood pressure.

Tapping - the insertion of a needle to drain off abnormal collections of fluid.

Temporal lobes - the lowermost parts of the cerebral hemispheres.

Tetanus - an infection which causes severe spasm in all groups of muscles.

Trachea - the wind-pipe.

Trephine - an instrument used to bore a hole in the skull.

Trigeminal neuralgia - an illness characterised by brief but recurrent bouts of intense pain in one side of the face.

Tropical sprue - chronic inflammation of the intestines with associated malnutrition.

Tuberculoma - a lump produced by a low-grade tuberculous infection.

The Yorkshire Medical and Dental History Society holds meetings – usually at the Thackrah Medical Museum, St. James's Hospital, Leeds – about six times a year. Details can be obtained from the Secretary, Mr. W. K. Mathie (Tel. 0113 233 4363).